Essential Mechanisms in Neurological Pediatric Rehabilitation

Ass. Prof. Dr. Ahmed Azzam

Department of Physiotherapy for
Developmental Disturbance and Pediatric
Surgery, Faculty of Physical Therapy,
Cairo University

Department of rehabilitation science, Faculty of
applied medical science
King saud university
2019

ISBN
978-1-5437-5010-2 (sc)
978-1-5437-5011-9 (e)

Library of Congress Control Number: 2019935855

Print information available on the last page.

To order additional copies of this book, contact
Toll Free 800 101 2657 (Singapore)
Toll Free 1 800 81 7340 (Malaysia)
www.partridgepublishing.com/singapore
orders.singapore@partridgepublishing.com

03/06/2019

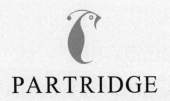

PARTRIDGE

<u>Contents</u>

Chapter 4
Syndromes in pediatric rehabilitation

Chapter 5
Human genetics

Chapter 6
(Developmental psychology)

Chapter 7
References (for further reading)

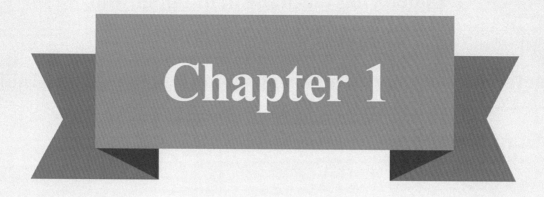

Chapter 1

Introduction

1-Underlying mechanism of upper and lower motor neuron lesion:

Characteristics of upper and lower motor neuron lesion: Table (1)

Characteristics of UMNL-LMNL	Upper motor neuron lesion	Lower motor neuron lesion
1-Paralysis -Extend -Side -Type -Recovery	-wide spread -opposite side -spastic -no recovery theoretically But recovery occur under umbrella of neural plasticity	-localized -same side -flaccid -complete recovery in neuro-praxia Incomplete recovery in axonotemeses No-recovery of neurotemeses
2-Muscle tone	Hypertonia (spastic, Rigidity, fluctuating hypertonia) Inhibitory tracts from cortex and corpus striatum are damaged but facilitatory vestibule-spinal and reticulo-spinal are working	Hypotonia (mild, moderate ,flaccidity) Due to reflex arch is damaged
3-Reflexes -Superficial reflexes -Deep reflexes	-lost as abdominal reflex - as babinski sign extension big toe due to pyramidal tract lesion+ fanning of other toes due to extra pyramidal tract lesion -hyper-reflexia	-lost as abdominal reflex -In partial lesion flexion of all toes occur -In complete lesion lost of response occur -hypo-reflexia
4-Wasting of muscle	-no wasting except with neglection(disuse atrophy)	- marked atrophy occur due to reflex arch is interrupted lead to loss of pumping action of muscle lead to protein catabolism inside muscle (sarcomere) decrease the muscle contour
5-Response to electric stimulation	-normal response to electric stimulation	-reaction of degeneration occur in LMNL due to complete cut of reflex arch(in ability to respond to electrical stimulation)
6-Blood supply and metabolism	-normal response	-decreased due to interruption of reflex arch

2-Underlying mechanism of spasticity:

The pyramidal system consists of pyramidal tracts which is facilitatory to muscle tone and extra-pyramidal tracts which has facilitatory and inhibitory tracts making a balance between facilitation and inhibition to muscle tone producing smooth movment. In stroke there is cerebral artery disorder either occlusion or hemorrhage causing interruption of blood supply to the pyramidal system leading to loss of the inhibitory impulses of extra pyramidal tracts and facilitatory impulses of both pyramidal and extra pyramidal tracts except two facilitatory vestibule-spinal and reticulo-spinal tracts which synapses with gamma and alpha motor neurons of stretch reflex leading to hypertonia and clumsy movement due to loss of reciprocal inhibition mechanism.

3-Underlying mechanism of atrophy:

Reflex arch is interrupted lead to loss of pumping action of muscle lead to protein catabolism inside muscle (sarcomere) decrease the muscle contour.

4-Underlying mechanism of hypotonia:

Reflex arch is damaged

5-Underlying mechanism of recovery in upper motor neuron lesion:

Never occur theoretically because tracts and nerve cells never regenerate but recovery can occur under the umbrella of neural plasticity.

Neural plasticity
1-Denervation super- sensitivity:
Denervation of part of organs stimulates the healthy part to increase its efficiency to compensate the degenerated part.

2-Resolution of odema:

Efficiency of venous system and villi is responsible for decreasing of central edema gradually

3-Diachasis:

The neighbor cells of degenerated cells are shocked (no organic lesion) loss its function temporary. After 2-6 weeks recovery occurred of the shocked cells and actually improvement appear on the patients

4-Axonal sprouting:

Motor neuron is regenerated by sprouting from 1-4 mm every day

5-Collateral sprouting:

Alternating routes occur to reach the healthy dendrites by healthy branches of axon and opposite to exclude the dead cell.

6-Unmasking of silent synapse:

Brain contains more than 33 trillion cells. Not all of them are actively participated. The function is occupied by competition in two ways either new skill or after lesion and dead of some cells so silent synapses become active and unmasking occur.

<u>6-Underlying mechanism of recovery in lower motor neuron lesion</u>

Factors affecting on prognosis of peripheral nerve lesion :

a-Age: The earlier of age the more chance of good recovery

b- Site of lesion: Proximal lesion is worse in prognosis than distal lesion

c-Extend of lesion: The more extends of lesion the worse in prognosis

Type of nerve lesion

1-**Neuropraxia:** Is physiological block of signals as a result of ischemia. Complete recovery occur spontaneously through 2 weeks

2-**Axonotemeses:** Interruption occurs through axon and myelin sheath but Schwan's cell is intact which is responsible for regeneration of myelin sheath the tube of the nerve regeneration so incomplete recovery occurs. Recover occur 3- 6months .Measure distance from lesion till the end of nerve then multiplied by 10(nerve regenerate from 1-4mm in day)

3-**Neurotemeses:** Interruption occurs through axon and myelin sheath in addition to Schwan's cell is dead so no recovery occur and flail limb is the result.

d-Associated lesion: Vessels lesion, dislocations and fractures delay the improvement.

e-Gap and severity of lesion: The more the gap between proximal and distal parts the more worse of prognosis.

f-Type of nerve fiber: The first nerve regenerate is the sensory nerve then motor then mixed nerve.

g-Area of sensory loss: The more area of sensory loss occurs after lesion the worse of prognosis.

7- Underlying mechanism of wide spread paralysis of UMNL

Pyramidal tracts are compact fiber any interruption lead to extend paralysis.

8- Underlying mechanism of Babinski sign

- Pathological Babinski sign: occur in UMNL, under anesthesia and coma (extension big toe due to pyramidal tract lesion and fanning of other toes due to extra pyramidal tract lesion) this positive response is normal in first year after that indicate to UMNL.
- Physiological Babinski sign: occur in deep sleep

9- Underlying mechanism of reaction of degeneration

- Occur in LMNL due to complete cut of reflex arch (in ability to respond to electrical stimulation)
- Did not occur in UMNL due to reflex arch is not interrupted (respond to electric stimulation)

10 -Underlying mechanism of quick stretch

quick stretch occur lead to stimulate gamma fibers lead to stimulate contractile part of intra-fusal muscle fiber lead to stimulate non contractile part which include stretch receptors sending afferent signals to PHC Then to AHC then to alpha motor neuron causing contraction of extra-fusal muscle fibers.

11- Underlying mechanism of prolonged stretch

For example: Prolonged stretch to hip adductor muscle to gain relaxation via: At first quick stretch occur leads to stimulate gamma fibers lead to stimulate contractile part of intra-fusal muscle fiber lead to stimulate non contractile part which include stretch receptors sending afferent signals to PHC Then to AHC then to alpha motor neuron causing contraction of extra-fusal muscle fibers. At second step just one contraction or repeated contraction occurred stimulate GTO sending 1b afferent to PHC then to 1b inter neuron which reverse the stimulated signals into inhibitory signals which inhibit AHC then inhibit alpha motor neuron then relaxate extra-fusal muscle fibers. Techniques used as prolonged stretch (positioning, night splint, reflex inhibiting pattern, Bobath technique) all of them depend on prolonged stretch.

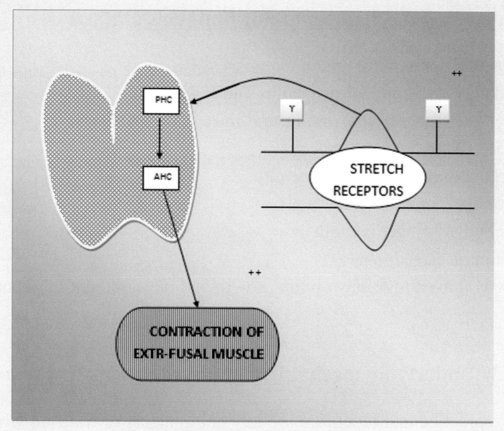

Fig (1): Quick stretch mechanism

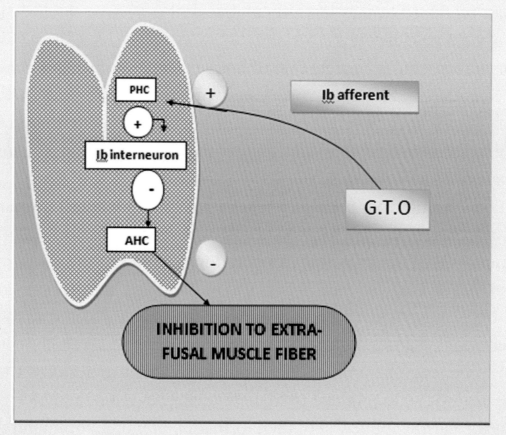

Fig (2): Prolonged stretch mechanism

12- Underlying mechanism of ant-fontanels clinical significance:

- Pre-mature closure: as in cranio -stenosis
- Delayed closure: as in hydrocephalus and rickets
- Bulging: as in hemorrhage (increase if intra cranial tension)
- Retracting: as in dehydration
- Measured at birth by 3 finger breadth
- At 6 months 2finger breadth
- At 12 months 1 finger breadth
- At 18 months closed
- One method used to follow up the growth and development to neonates and infant

13- Underlying mechanism of physiotherapy training

The more practice and repetition are key components of training which lead to more sensory input, feedback and permanent changes as new strategies and motor plan produced lead to learning a new skill or restore the lost skill. The nervous system provide the:

1. Sensory processing for perception of body orientation in space provided by visual, vestibular, and somato-sensory systems.
2. Sensory-motor integration essential for linking sensation to motor responses (centrally programmed postural adjustments that precede voluntary movement).
3. Mechanism of new motor strategy:

Information coming from periphery reached to the spinal cord through spinal nerves, information coming from head and neck reached to brainstem through cranial nerves. All the previous information reached to the thalamus to be sensitized then to the post-central gyrus to be localized. Perception, cognition, new sensory strategy will be produced by sensory areas which lead to increase of efficiency of synapses. After that information reach to cerebellum and basal ganglion to be smoothening and prevention of excessive activity, then reach to pre-central gyrus to produce permanent changes and new motor behavior. Which mean learning of new skill then formation of motor command via tracts to final common pathway (alpha and gamma MN) to perform new behavior of skills or reacquisition of fine and gross motor skill.

14-Underlying mechanism of pyramidal and extra-pyramidal tracts: Table: (2)

Pyramidal T	Extrapyramidal T
1-Only one neuron from cortex to A.H.Cs without synapse	1-multiple neurons from cortex to AHCs with many synapse
2-Occupies pyramid of medulla	2-don't occupy the pyramid
3-Origin localized(area 4) and area 8	3-origin wide(all cortical areas with area 6 on top
4-85% of fibers cross to opposite side at pyramide15 % cross at cervical level	4-some tracts cross and others don't
5-Doesnot function in first year of life(not yet mylinated)i.e. undeveloped	5-function in first year of life
6-Facilitatory to muscle tone and deep reflexes (pure lesion decrease tone and reflexes). pure lesion occur at area 4 only	6-some tracts are facilitatory but others inhibitory. Lesion lead to increase tone and reflexes
7-Responsible for fine isolated and skillful movements as in hand function(grasping, voluntary release, eye hand co ordination, hand manipulative skills, bilateral hand use, reaching) It initiates voluntary movements	7-responsible for gross movement using large groups of muscles As (sitting skills, swinging arm during walking) They coordinate voluntary movements

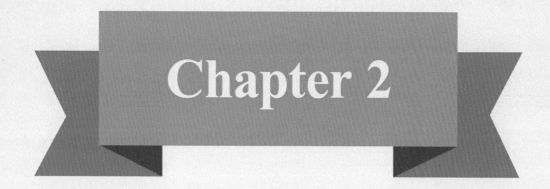

Chapter 2

Lower Motor Neuron Diseases

- Brachial plexus injury (Erb's palsy- klumpks paralysis- whole arm type)
- Facial palsy

Brachial plexus injury (Erb's palsy- klumpks paralysis- whole arm type):

1-Underlying mechanism of brachial plexus injury:

- Erb's palsy: forced lateral flexion of neck against fixed shoulder
- Klumpks paralysis: forced upward movement or forced abduction of shoulder
- Whole arm type: avulsion of brachial plexus roots from the cord or neurotemeses type of nerve lesion→ flail limb

2- Underlying mechanism of Erb's point stimulation:

- It is the six meeting nerves point (C5, C6 Roots-anterior and posterior divisions nerve to sub-clavius and supra-scapular nerve)
- It is the point for electric stimulation for upper limb
- It is the point for probe laser application for nerve proliferation
- It is located at the lower 1/3 of sternoclidomastoid muscle just behind clavicle

3- Underlying mechanism of proximal and distal lesion in Erb's palsy:

- The more proximal to the roots the more worse of prognosis
- Proximal lesion may include of root lesion leading to winging of scapula due to paralysis of serratus anterior and rhomboid which supplied from roots C5, 6,7
- It can be located by observe the winging of the scapula or by measure the distance between medial border of the scapula and spine on both sides. it increased on winging side
- Distal lesion has good prognosis due to scapula is free from lesion and decrease the extend of paralysis

4-Underlying mechanism of Erb's engram:

- Appear in recovery stage the middle fiber of deltoid is innervated before anterior fiber so when the child makes reaching he makes abduction instead of flexion of shoulder

- It can be prevented before sitting by training the child to reach the object by flexion of shoulder also we can use the wall to prevent abduction during reaching and use flexion

Physical problems of Erb's engram:
1-Paralysis of anterior fiber of deltoid
2-Tightness of biceps brachii
3-Lmitation of scapular movement
4-Bad habits of abduction shoulder during reaching

Treatment of Erb's engram:
1-Facilitatory techniques +functional electrical stimulation for anterior fiber of deltoid

2-Passive stretching for bicep brachii via abduction of shoulder90 + supination of forearm+ wrist extension
- Stretch to long head of biceps brachii via cupping of shoulder at edge of bed the extension of elbow with wrist extension and gradually hyper-extend of shoulder till pain appear then sustain 20 second and rest 20second

3-Scapular mobilization:
Scapular mobilization is performed from side lying position facing to physiotherapist, the index hold medial border of scapula, thumb hold lateral border of scapula and web space hold inferior angle of scapula, then perform mobilization in upward rotation and down ward rotation, adduction the abduction of scapula. Sets of 10 repetitions were applied with a rest interval of 30 seconds between sets. The intervention consisted of applying superior and inferior gliding, rotations, and distraction to the scapula of the affected shoulder. The participants laid the affected forearm on their back. The therapist stood before

the patient's affected shoulder, placing the index finger of one hand under the medial scapular border, the other hand grasping the superior border of the scapula. The scapula was moved superiorly and inferiorly for superior and inferior glide, and then the scapula was rotated upward and downward for scapular rotation.

Second, with the patient was in the same position the physiotherapist put the ulnar fingers under the medial -scapular border and distracted the scapula from the thorax. These patterns were chosen because decreases in scapular upward rotation, posterior tilt, superior tilt, and external rotation.

The third technique shoulder joint gliding with scapular mobilization from side lying position backed to physiotherapist the thumb hold medial border of scapula, index hold shoulder in completely adduction and resting on trunk the apply upward rotation of scapula with superior gliding and downward rotation of scapula with inferior gliding, then retraction of scapula with posterior gliding of shoulder and protraction of scapula with anterior gliding of shoulder. Sets of 10 repetitions were applied with a rest interval of 30 seconds between sets.

At last shoulder manipulation the child in side lying backed to physio-therapist,one hand of physiotherapist fix scapula and the otherhand perform adduction of shoulder with gradual flexion in shoulder which perform stretch on posterior capsule of shoulder repeat 3 times for 5 times maximum with a rest interval of 30 seconds between sets. 4-correct the abnormal engram manually by fix scapula by one hand and ask child to make adduction of shoulder with extension of elbow with repetition.

5- Underlying mechanism of catching engram:

- It appear in recovery stage due to weakness of wrist extensors, tightness of wrist flexors and pronators + abnormal attitude (pronation of forearm+ wrist flexion/P flexion finger extension) during feeding and ADL activities

Physical problems of catching engram:
1-Weakness of wrist extensors
2-Tightness of wrist flexors

3-Tightness of pronators and loss of supination

4-Abnorma attitude during feeding and ADL

Treatment of catching engram:

1-Facilitatory techniques to wrist extensors+ faradic stimulation to wrist extensors

2-Passive stretch to wrist flexors manually + positioning as quadruped + hand weight bearing ex.

3-Passive stretching of pronators +facilitation of supination

Specific treatment suggestions for enhancing supination:

1-Encourage mouthing and finger feeding

2-Facilitate supination with the forearm on a surface as in weight bearing on floor, or on mat,while seated at a table the therapist place an object in the child hand,the child attempt to compensate for difficulty with supination by using wrist extension

3-Encourage the use of 45 to 90 degrees of supination followed by grasp of an object with elbow in 90 degrees of flexion,the child encourage to keep thumb up as reaching and grasping large birthday candles then put them into cake that require supination

4-Encourage lateral reach followed by grasp most of children with limited use of supination find it easier to combine humeral abduction with external rotation and supination than to use humeral flexion with external rotation and supination. Object presented laterally to the child allow the child to use abduction and external rotation which allow for supination

5-Encourage reaching by using shoulder flexion and external rotation by placing the object between leg and shoulder in sitting position depending on the child ability to control external rotation and supination while completing the reach.

6-Encourage reaching across midline following strategies suggested for reaching in front of the shoulder.

7-Correct the abnormal attitude via supination of forearm + wrist extension+ training of finger flexion on an object then extension with repetition.

6-Under lying mechanism of neuro-muscular electrical stimulation in Erb's palsy children:

The electrical stimulation inhibited increases in all 3 protein degradation pathways linked to atrophied serratus anterior and stimulate protein synthesis (increase number of sarcomere) inside muscle so it can be used to treat and prevent muscle atrophy skeletal muscle atrophy is characterized by decrease protein synthesis and increased protein degradation. the decrease in protein synthesis reaches a peak within a few days after the start of unloading whereas the increase in protein degradation reaches a peak 14 days after unloading it was hypothesized that the increase in protein degradation was related closely rather than the decrease in protein synthesis to the atrophied muscle three major protein degradation pathways are implicated in skeletal muscle atrophy resulting from a variety of disuse conditions (e.g., unloading, immobilization, denervation) it can be postulated that the decreases in muscle mass and muscle fiber cross-sectional areas in muscles were due to the activation of the 3 major protein degradation pathways .

Denervated muscles had an abnormal structural appearance myofibrils were thinner and fewer in number and they were often discontinuous sarcomeres lacked M-line or showed streaming of Z-lines and the registration normally seen across the fiber was lost. wide spaces between the myofibrils were filled with amorphous cyto skeletal material. mitochondrial function may have been disrupted by the loss of their normal distribution and structural associations within the fibers and fragments of the sarcoplasmic reticulum and T system.

The flaccid paralysis that result from these LMNL has more serious consequences the muscles lose mass rapidly and much of the cross section become occupied by non contractile tissue notably collagen and fat.

7-Under lying mechanism of scapular mobilization in improvement of shoulder flexion:

End-of-range passive movements may reduce peripheral input to the CNS, thereby decreasing pain, in two ways. The first is via a temporary reduction in intra-articular pressure due to decreased tension on the joint capsule and inhibition of muscle contraction by discharge produced in joint afferents with end of joint mobilization movement. This decrease in tension could be due either to fluid reduction within the joint space or to stretch of collagen fibrils.

The second way in which end-of-range passive movements may reduce peripheral input to the CNS is through adaptation of the encapsulated endings of joint nerves to the mechanical stimulus of prolonged stretch of the peri-articular soft tissue. Secondary effects of improved mobility include beneficial effects on joint cartilage and improved blood and lymphatic flow. Passive motion has demonstrated significant increases in cellularity, cell products, strength, and mobility in those tissues receiving passive motion.

A possible mechanism for this increase in range may be the improved nutrition of cartilage produced by movement, improved matrix organization, collagen concentration, strength, and linear stiffness of ligament scars that were moved in immobilization Joint Mobilization Is a type of passive movement performed by the PT at a speed slow enough that the patient can stop the movement. The tech. may be applied with Oscillatory motion TO ↓Pain and (or) ↑mobility.

All can be treated with gentle joint play technique to stimulate neuro-physiological and mechanical effects.
- Neuro-physiological effect: Small amplitude oscillatory move→ stimulate mechano-receptor → ↓ transmission of nociceptive stimuli via stimulate theories of pain.
- Mechanical effects: Small-amplitude movement → synovial fluid motion→ bring nutrients to the vascular portions of articular cartilage (↓ischemia) .

- Gentle joint play → maintain nutrient exchange → prevent painful effects of stasis when a joint is painful or swollen and can't move through a ROM. (but not in acute or massive swelling).

8-Under lying mechanism of developmental considerations during mobilization:

There are a number of neuro-developmental disabilities for which joint Mobilization and particularly spinal manipulation, would be strongly Contra indicated. Although physical therapists would likely not use joint mobilization in the presence of hyper mobile joints, specific statements about the children for whom this treatment is contraindicated are warranted.

In the child with pure athetoid and ataxic forms of cerebral palsy, joints tend to be hypermobile. hypermobility of the spine in children with athetoid cerebral palsy may lead to cervical instability; researchers have noted that "rapid and repetitious neck movements seem to accelerate the progression of cervical instability in athetoid CP patients."

Another common neuro-developmental disability in which joints are hyper-mobile secondary to lax ligaments is Down syndrome. In a report of *265*individuals with Down syndrome, 23% of the subjects had patellar instability leading to sub-luxation or dislocation and 10% had hip sub-luxation or dislocation.51 Of even greater concern in Down Syndrome is the presence of atlanto-axial instability, which has been reported in up to 15% of individuals with this disorder.52 Other, less common, neuro-developmental disabilities, such as Prader- WilliSyndrome, may be characterized by generalized Hypotonia and hyper mobile joints. For these children as well, joint mobilizationWould be contra-indicated.

Many children with generalized development delay of unknown etiology also exhibit hypotonia and ligamentous laxity. In the typically developing child, somatic muscle growth is stimulated by skeletal growth as a result of the increasing distance imposed on the muscle attachments as bone grows. Thus, skeletal muscles "increase in length in parallel with, and apparently in response to, bone growth. Such changes in muscle may develop if opposing muscles are paralyzed or weak, as in the case of the child with Erb's palsy or in a child with hypotonia.

When the agonist muscle fails to grow normally, muscle tightness result. Similarly, changes in muscle can have an effect on bones or joints (e.g., muscle tightness will lead to a decrease in joint movement with possible subsequent conversion of part of the articular cartilage into fibrous tissue). Growth cartilage is present at three sites in the developing child: the Epiphyseal plate, the joint surface, and the apophysis or tendon insertion Injuries to each of these sites as a result of the repetitive stresses.

The predisposition of immature growth plates to injury-particularly during growth spurts suggests the need to be cautious when using joint mobilization in children. Although muscle and bone growth are delayed in the involved limbs of children with Erb's palsy growth spurts presumably take place, because overall growth occurs. Paralyzed muscle grows more slowly than normal muscle in relation to bone growth the musculoskeletal development of children with Erb's palsy is different from typically developing children. alterations in bone and muscle growth occur as a result of the effect of prolonged paralysis movement restriction in older children with long-standing hypo-mobility may be secondary to capsular tightening and adhesions inaddition to muscle tightness.

Joint mobilization in conjunction with neuro-physiological forms of therapeutic exercise, may be indicated for such children. Cautions however, that capsular dysfunction may be difficult to differentiate from movement restriction caused by muscle tightness. The capsular changes seen in adhesive capsulitis have been described as a "gluing together" of the synovial surfaces in the pouched area of the capsule. This portion of the capsule becomes thickened and contracted; the synovial fluid becomes more viscous, and the walls of the capsule adhere to each other. These capsular changes prohibit the downward movement of the humerus in the glenoid fossa during abduction and forward flexion. Even when positioning and handling are used to inhibit increased tone and facilitate movement, joint ROM may remain limited because of Capsular tightening.

Inferior shoulder capsule tightness might affect shoulder flexion and abduction, because the scapulo-thoracic joint is composed by muscles, not like synovial joints. SM may break up adhesions and release these muscles; hence, scapular movement may be increased. The improvement of shoulder movement might also be related to increased scapular movement.

It is accepted that the gleno-humeral and scapula-thoracic joints are in the enclosed kinetic chain. We assume that if gleno-humeral mobilization improves shoulder movements and normalizes the scapula-humeral rhythm, scapular mobilization should improve shoulder movements; this is related with our endings, because of the relation between shoulder and scapular.

Joint-mobilization techniques also have neurophysiologic effects, which are based on the stimulation of peripheral mechanoreceptors and the inhibition of nociceptors. These mechanoreceptors are present mostly around synovial joint. Synovial joint mobilization may provide sufficient sensory input to activate the endogenous pain-inhibitory systems. Scapular mobilization maybe related to muscle structures rather than the synovial joint, which is rich in mechanoreceptors. Shoulder flexion function after the application of SM. Our primary interest was to assess SM related to shoulder ROM and shoulder-function disabilities. When scapular and shoulder movements are improved, shoulder functional status gets better.

9-Underlying mechanism of weight bearing ex . In Erb's palsy:

- Proprioceptive training (static and dynamic stimulation)
- Increase muscle pull produce powerful contraction
- Stimulate bone growth (prevent delaying of bone growth)
- Increase cross section of bone (deposition of ca on bone)
- Increase cross section of muscle (stimulate anabolism inside muscle)
- Stimulate reciprocal movement between upper limbs
- Stimulate normal reciprocal inhibition and normal co contraction between agonist and antagonist

10-Underlying mechanism of serratus anterior stimulation in proximal lesion of Erb's palsy:

The scapula is the largest bone of the shoulder complex and has the greatest number of muscles attached to it these muscles both stabilize the arm to the body and move the arm around in space all these muscles act at the same time sometimes and oppose each other at other times but work together like a well trained team to allow the arm to move in space if any of these muscles are not working in the right way at the right time this leads to a break in the rhythmic motion of the scapula winged scapula is a common biomechanical deficiency which is caused by loss of serratus anterior muscle function loss of trapezius muscle function weakness of all the scapula winging secondary to instability winging secondary to brachial plexus injury the serratus anterior muscle is also known as the boxers muscle because that is one of the motions it does it protracts (or brings the shoulder forward) if this muscle is weak it does not hold the scapula as close to the ribcage and the result of that is called winging .
Scapular winging has been observed to disrupt scapula-humeral rhythm contributing to decreased flexion and abduction of the upper extremity as well as a loss in power and the source of considerable pain the serratus anterior muscle attaches to the medial anterior aspect of the scapula (i.e.it attaches on the side of the scapula that faces the ribcage)and normally anchor the scapula against the rib cage when the serratus anterior contracts upward rotation abduction and weak elevation of the scapula occurs allowing the arm to be raised above the head the long thoracic nerve innervates the serratus anterior therefore damage to or impingement of the muscle if this occurs the scapula may slip away from the rib cage giving it the wing-like appearance on the upper back this characteristic may particularly be seen when the affected person pushes against resistance

Serratus anterior muscles cannot be stimulated effectively except in winging of scapula as in proximal lesion of Erb's palsy due to the appearance of its fibers in addition to traditional physiotherapy program as above the electrical stimulation apparatus with two channels electrical were applied on rhomboid-deltoid technique for improving normal scapular rotation the subject was enrolled in a day after day stimulation continue for 15 minutes with 70 HZ pulse width of 300 microsecond stimulation of the muscles surrounding the scapula for the purpose of stabilization during other joint movements may be desirable although activation of the middle trapezius and rhomboid muscles may achieve a degree of scapular adduction winging of the scapula generally is not resolved without stimulation of the serratus anterior muscle the patient demonstrating serratus anterior

Muscle weakness and secondary scapular winging can use electrical stimulation for facilitation as when a scapula has separated from the rib cage sufficiently so that an electrode can be placed over the ventral aspect of scapular surface a second electrode may be placed on the lower lateral side of the trunk or one electrode under the winged scapula and the second electrode over the broad area of the serratus anterior muscles origin stimulation can provide adequate realignment of the scapula to correct its winged posture as the patient gains strength in the serratus anterior muscle and the winging of the scapula becomes less pronounced placement of the electrode becomes increasingly difficult after the scapula is repositioned appropriately on the trunk and no longer wings achieving further realignment of the scapula with electrical stimulation may be difficult or even impossible we have been unsuccessful in activating the serratus anterior muscle unless we can position the a electrode over the ventral (anterior) surface of the scapula .

The serratus anterior is a broad flattened sheet of muscle originating from the first nine ribs and passes posteriorly around the thoracic wall before inserting into the costal surface of the medial border of the scapula the serratus anterior has three functional components the superior component originates from the first and second ribs and inserts into the superior medial angle of the scapula this component serves as the scapula this component serves as the anchor that allows the scapula to rotate when the arm is lifted overhead the middle component of the serratus anterior originates from the third fourth and fifth ribs and inserts on the vertebral border of the scapula serving to protract the scapula the inferior component originates from the sixth to ninth ribs and inserts on the inferior angle of the scapula this third portion serves to protract the scapula and rotate the inferior angle upward and laterally as a whole the main function of the serratus anterior is to protract and rotate the scapula keeping it closely opposed to the thoracic wall and optimizing the position of the glenoid for maximum efficiency for upper extremity motion

The serratus anterior is solely innervated by the long thoracic nerve (C5,C6,and C7) originating from the anterior rami of the fifth sixth and seventh cervical nerves branches from the fifth and sixth cervical nerves pass anteriorly through the scalenus medius muscle before joining the seventh cervical nerve branch that coursed anteriorly to the scalenus medius the long thoracic nerve then dives deep to the brachial plexus and the clavicle to pass over the first rib here the nerve enters a fascial sheath and continues to descend along the lateral aspect of the thoracic wall to innervate the serratus anterior muscle .

11-Underlying mechanism of different types of brachial plexus injuries:

Comparison between different types of brachial plexus lesion Table: (3)

Characteristics	Erbs palsy	Klumpks paralysis	Whole arm type
1-Site of lesion	Upper trunk(C5-C6) If C7 involved paralysis of elbow extensors and wrist extensor occur.If C4 involved unilateral paralysis of diaphragm occur.	Lower trunk(C8-T1) If T2 involved Homer syndrome occur	Whole plexus can be involved
2-Mechanism of injury	forced lateral flexion of neck against fixed shoulder	forced upward movement or forced abduction of shoulder	avulsion of brachial plexus roots from the cord or neurotemeses type of nerve lesion→ flail limb
3-Cyanosis and irregular respiration	Occur if C4 involved in lesion (immediately after birth)	Don't occur(away from C4)	Occur if C4 involved
4-Paralysed muscles	-ant ,middle and posterior fibers of deltoid	-flexors and extensors of the	-paralysis of all muscles of

		wrist	UL
	-biceps brachii -supinator	-intrinsic muscles of the hand	
5-Tight muscles	-sub-scapularis -pronators -wrist flexors -peri- scapular muscles(if the lesion is proximal) -in recovery stage biceps brachii involved in tightness	-as a result of gravity tightness of wrist flexors and intrinsic muscles of hand	Flail limb
6-Attitude of limb	-porter tip hand -policeman tip position Extension, adduction, and internal rotation of shoulder with elbow extension and pronation of forearm If C7 involved wrist flexors tightness and ulnar deviation occur	-claw hand due to gravity	Flail limb
7-Sensory loss	As a coin shape on lateral aspect of arm	Medial side of arm, medial side of forearm And palmar 3 and half fingers and 1.5 dorsal finger	Whole sensations are lost

8-Scapular involvement	-Involved if the lesion is proximal -free with distal lesion	-don't involved	-involved
9-Proximal or distal dysfunction	-mainly proximal affection	-mainly distal affection	-both proximal and distal affection
10-Horner syndrome	-do not present	present	present
11-Type of nerve lesion	-neuro praxia or -axonotemeses	-neuro praxia or -axonotemeses	neurotemeses
12-Physical problem	-paralysis of muscles(as above) -tightness of muscles(as above) -sensory loss(as above) -shortening of the limb -atrophy -peri-scapular adhesions -adhesions of shoulder posterior capsule -in recovery stage: Erb engram, catch engram and tightness of biceps brachii	-paralysis of muscles(as above) -tightness of muscles(as above) -loss of hand functions -sensory loss(as above)	- whole paralysis and sensation lost

13-Treatment	-faradic stimulation to stimulate protein synthesis inside muscle(sarcomere)→prevent and treat atrophy -weight bearing ex. On hand(prevent and treat shortening of limb) -facilitation of muscle contraction -Proprioceptive training -scapular mobilization -gleno-humeral mobilization -balance training -stretching of tight muscles -manage erb and catch engram -fastening clothes of the arm with forearm(positioning)	-reciprocate stimulation for flexors and extensors of wrist(stimulate reciprocal inhibition of agonist and antagonist) --weight bearing ex. On hand(prevent and treat shortening of limb) -facilitation of muscle contraction proprioceptive training -balance training -stretching of tight muscles -night wrist splint	-the same treatment as in erbs for 3 months and followed by NCV -Decision making if discharged or not
14-Recovery and prognosis	Neuro-praxia→good prognosis(complete recovery) axonotemeses→good prognosis(incomplete recovery)	-the same	Neurotemeses (no recovery)

12-Underlying mechanism of facilitatory techniques used in LMN diseases:

1)-Quick stretch

Stimulation of gamma fibers via (quick stretch on muscle or motor command) lead to stimulate contractile part of intra-fusal muscle fiber lead to stimulate non contractile part which include stretch receptors(flower spray and annulo-spiral receptors) sending afferent(Ia) signals to PHC. Then to AHC then to alpha motor neuron causing contraction of extra-fusal muscle fibers.

2) - Tapping followed by movement

Tapping on muscle belly will produce quick elongation of muscle fiber→ stimulate gamma fibers produce contraction of muscle

3) - Resistance for strong muscle firing motor neuron pool of weak muscle

Use the strong muscles to produce irradiation firing to motor neuron pool of weak muscles

4) - High frequency vibration

Fast vibration will stimulate sensory afferent nerve (Ia) produce muscle contraction

5) -Approximation (proprioceptive stimulation):

Static and dynamic approximation will stimulate static and dynamic proprioceptors in and around joint→sensory feedback→dorsal Colum tracts→feeling in thalamus → localized in post-central gyrus →remodeling and smoothening by cerebellum→prevent excessive activity by basal ganglion→modulated in pre-central gyrus→motor command by modulation of muscle tone

6)-Repetitive brushing

Repetitive brushing→ Extro-ceptive stimulation →sensory feed back (one method of sensory integration therapy)

7) -Biofeed back

Visual and auditory feedback→stimulate motivation effect on the children→activation of muscles

8) - Electric stimulation

In atrophy we are in a bad need for electric stimulation to stimulate the protein synthesis inside muscle which was decreased in atrophy.
Electric stimulation produce depolarization of the skin which transferred to nerve stimulate sensory nerve first then with increase power will stimulate motor fiber produce muscle contraction

9) -Weight bearing

- Proprioceptive training (static and dynamic stimulation)

- Increase muscle pull produce powerful contraction
- Stimulate bone growth (prevent delaying of bone growth)
- Increase cross section of bone (deposition of ca on bone)
- Increase cross section of muscle (stimulate anabolism inside muscle)
- Stimulate reciprocal movement between upper limbs
- Stimulate normal reciprocal inhibition and normal co contraction between agonist and antagonist

10) - Vestibular stimulation:
- Static labyrinth: stimulated by linear acceleration and vertical movement→utricle and saccula→tilting of cupula→++vestibulo-cochlear nerve→vestibulo-spinal tract→modulate alpha motor neuron→modulate muscle tone
- Dynamic labyrinth: stimulated by angular acceleration (rotation)→stimulate endo- lymph in semicircular canal→++vestibulo-cochlear nerve→vestibulo-spinal tract→modulate alpha motor neuron→modulate muscle tone

11) - Brief icing
- ++of gamma fibers→contraction of muscle

12) -Extroceptive stimulation:
- Clenching toes+ painful stimuli on sole of foot and tibial plateau +rabbing +firm pressure on shaft of tibia →stimulation to muscle contraction

Facial palsy

12-Underlying mechanisms of phenomenas in facial palsy

-Bell's phenomena
During awaking eye ball move upward and laterally but we can't see it. In sleep we can see the eye ball move upward and laterally because the patient can't close his eye on the affected side.

-Crocodile tear phenomena

Wrong innervations occur when the lesion occur before geniculate ganglion the motor nerve of facial nerve regenerate in wrong pathway to supply the salivary and lachrymal gland which supplied by parasympathetic in normal condition. So when the patient laughs or eats or makes any motor action by face leading to tears

13-Underlying mechanism of paralysis distribution in upper and lower motor neuron facial palsy:

- Paralysis in upper motor neuron facial palsy takes opposite lower quarter of face because upper part of facial nucleus at Pons is bilaterally supplied by pyramidal tract but the lower part of the nucleus is unilaterally supplied
- Paralysis in lower motor neuron facial palsy take one half of the face due to interruption of reflex arch lead to upper and lower quarter of face on same side.

14-Underlying mechanism of crossed hemiplegia in Bells palsy:

Hemiplegia occur on opposite side of bell's palsy so crossed hemiplegia include(lower motor neuron bell's palsy on one side+ upper motor neuron facial included in hemiplegia on other side)

15-Underlying mechanism of facial expression in upper and lower motor neuron facial palsy:

Extra-pyramidal tracts responsible for the facial expression so the facial expression is free due to it is caused mainly from pyramidal tract lesion in UMNF and lost in LMNF due to interruption of reflex arch.

16-Underlying mechanism of facial muscles and skeletal muscles:

The facial muscles are subcutaneous (just under the skin) muscles that control facial expression. They generally originate from the surface of the skull bone (rarely the fascia), and insert on the skin of the face. When they contract, the skin moves. These muscles also cause wrinkles at right angles to the muscles' action line. Use of these muscles is noted during an extra- oral examination, assuring function of the nerve to these muscles

Comparison between facial muscles and skeletal muscles: Table: (4)

characteristics	Facial muscles	Skeletal muscles
Origin and insertion	originate from the surface of the skull bone (rarely the fascia), and insert on the skin of the face	Originate from bone and ends at bone
proprioceptors	Contain Less muscle spindle	Contain high number of muscle spindle
General function	Facial expression plus the specific function as press cheeks against teeth (buccinators)	-ROM -weight bearing -gait -endurance
Nerve supply	Cranial nerves	Spinal nerves

17-Underlying mechanism of causes of facial palsy:

1-Air draft→myositis→edema→compression on facial nerve→paralysis
2-Otitis media→due to viral or bacterial infection→inflammation→edema→ compression on facial nerve→paralysis
3-Congenital narrowing of stylo-mastoid foramen→ compression on facial nerve→paralysis

4-Diabetic, hypertension and atherosclerotic patient are more subjective to facial palsy.

5-Diabetic patient has high level of glucose in blood which transferred to sorbitol (alcohol) deposited on the nerve cells →peripheral neuritis→facial palsy

6-Atherosclerosis of the vasa nervosa will decrease of blood supply to facial nerve → peripheral neuritis→facial palsy

7-Hypertension →congestion of the nerve+ atherosclerosis→facial palsy

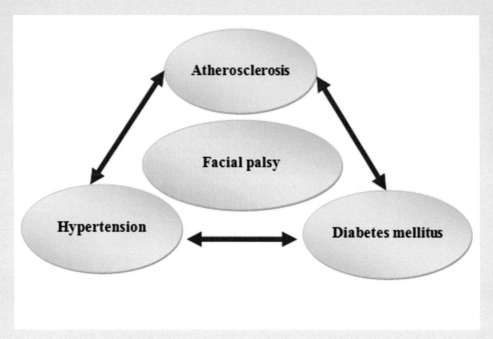

Fig (3): Predisposing factors of facial palsy

8-Deficiency of vit.B12 is an important cause of peripheral neuritis→facial palsy

9-Auto-immune cause →specific anti-body →attack the facial nerve→ facial palsy

10-Psychic causes

11-Burn and car accident

18-Underlying mechanism of UMNF and LMNF characteristics:

Comparison between UMNF and LMNF characteristics: Table: (5)

Characteristics	UMNF	LMNF
Site	Pyramidal tract lesion	Interruption of facial nerve
Side	Opposite side of lesion	Same side of lesion
Extend	Lower quarter of face	Half of the face
Fascial expression	intact	affected
Crossed hemiplegia	Must include with hemiplegia	If associated with hemiplegia called crossed hemiplegia
Muscle tone	Hypertonia	Hypotonia
Reflexes	Normal coroneal and glabellum reflex Hyper-reflexia of jaw reflex	Lost of blinking Hypo-reflexia of jaw reflex
Atrophy	Not present	present
Recovery	Associated with hemiplegia	According to type of nerve lesion(neuropraxia-axonotemeses-neurotemeses)

19-Underlying mechanism of pain in bell's palsy:

- Non suppurative inflammation through stylo-mastoid foramen (in- front, bellow and behind the ear)

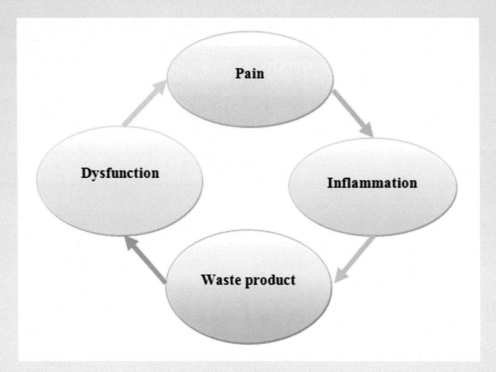

Fig (4): Underlying mechanism of pain and dysfunction in Bell's palsy

- The main anti- inflammatory method in physiotherapy is the short wave which produce deep heating removing the waste product and destroy the inflammation cycle

20-Underlying mechanism of adhesions in Bell's palsy:

- Improper function of muscles→forming adhesions inside muscles as in forehead muscles and zygomatic arch
- Friction manipulation on forehead and myo-facial release (pressure on zygomatic arch followed by release)

21-Underlying mechanism of mouth deviation in Bell's palsy:

Paralysis of mouth muscles on affected side → deviation of mouth toward the sound side due to imbalance between both sides

22-Underlying mechanism of treatment methods in Bell's palsy:

- Once there still pain around ear (in front-bellow-behind) continue with short wave diathermy is a must
- Once there is paralysis of facial muscles (zero muscle contraction) continue with faradic stimulation +passive movement followed by movement till muscle contraction gained then graduated active ex. Used and stop faradic stimulation
- Graduated active ex. Started by active assisted then after sharing of the child with ex. Transferred to active free ex. Then we can use irradiation of sound frontalis to make firing of motor neuron pool of the weak side
- PNF used by use maximum resistance to neck muscles extensors to facilitate the facial muscles which are directed upward. Maximum resistance to neck flexors can be used to facilitate the facial muscles in downward direction. Maximum resistance to lateral flexors of neck can be used to facilitate facial muscles in lateral direction
- Once deviation of mouth and opened eye still present continue with hand manipulation therapy for correction
- Probe laser therapy was used to facilitate the proliferation of ATP→facilitate regeneration of facial nerve
- Infra-red can be used on non-affected side for relaxation and improve circulation to prevent contracture
- Hock splint must be used after each session to gain new range of improved mouth deviation

N.B: Two wrong advices to Bell's palsy patients:

1- chewing of gum help in contraction of facial muscles (WRONG)
Because the masticatory muscles (supplied by trigeminal nerve) are responsible for chewing as a first step of swallowing
2- blowing of balloon is useful for facial muscle -contraction (WRONG) .Because blowing makes stretch on buccinators muscle →prolonged stretch→weakness→atrophy

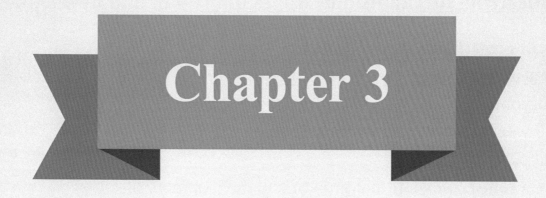

Chapter 3

Cerebral palsy

1-Underlying mechanism of stages of growth and development:

Stages of growth and development:

1)-Intra-uterine stage

a- Embryonic period:

First 12 weeks of pregnancy (organogenesis)

b- Fetal period:

1-Early: From 12-28wk (rapid growth and development of fetus)

2-Late: From28-40wk (period of further maturation of the featus)

2) Extra-uterine stage:

a-Neonatal period:

First 4 wk of life)adaptation with new life)

b- Infancy: First 2 years of life beyond neonatal period (most of rapid growth and development)

C-Childhood:

1-Early: From2-5y

2-Late: From5-12y

d- Adolescence: From 12-15ytransmission to a new adult

e-Early adulthood:From15-18yit end by union of the epiphysis

1-Underlying mechanism of reflexes:

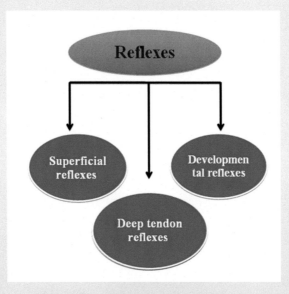

Fig (5): Types of reflexes

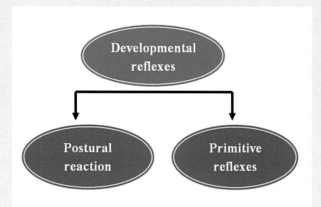

Fig (6): Reflexes responsible for CNS maturation

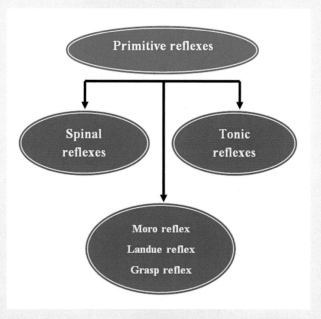

Fig (7): Sub- cortical inborn reflexes

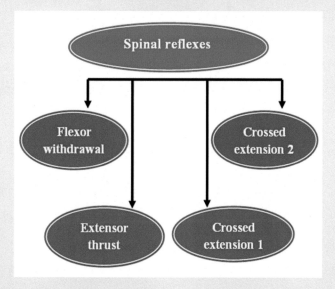

Fig (8): spinal inborn primitive reflexes

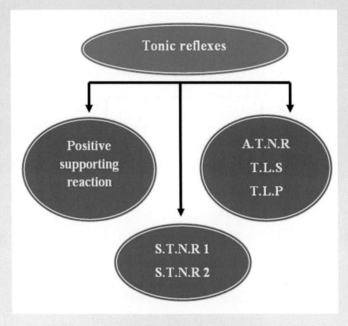

Fig (9): Pathological reflexes

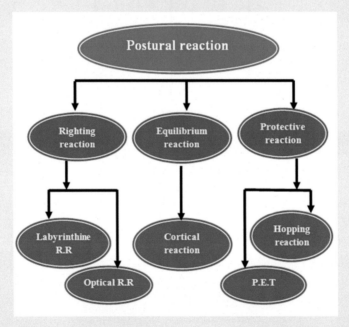

Fig (10): Acquired postural control reactions

2-Underlying mechanism of clinical importance of reflexes:

In new born infant, cerebral cortex is not developed so the CNS functions are carried out by the sub-cortical centers in the brainstem and spinal cord which mediate a number of primitive reflexes.

- when the infant grow the cerebral cortex develop and the higher center take up the functions of sub-cortical centers which lead to disappearance of primitive reflexes.

Value of primitive reflexes:

1-Their absence: during time they should be present indicate damage of the sub-cortical area concerned with the reflex

2-Their persistence: beyond the time they should disappear indicate failure of development of the cortical area that must suppress the reflex

Importance of reflexes:

1-Used as a diagnostic tool

2-Used as a method of facilitation of mile stone

3-Used as inhibition of abnormal pattern

Value of primitive reflexes: Table (6)

Reflex	Concern
Moro reflex: -Allow infant head to fall backward -sudden withdrawal of the blanket	1-normal reflex indicate normal CNS. 2-May signify cerebral birth injury if lacking or absence. -3-Asymmetric in erbs palsy. 4--exagegerated reflex indicate CNS irritation as jaundice 5-persistance after 4 months indicate cerebral palsy May indicate cerebral palsy or other neurological problem if persists past normal time.
-asymmetric tonic reflex -symetrical tonic neck 1,2 -tonic labyrinthine supine,prone -positive supporting reaction	

3-Underlying mechanism of newborn appearance

Types of newborn appearance:-
1-Normal appearance
2Hypotonia
3-Hypertonia
4-Hypotonia of back muscles
5-Opisthotonus

4-Underlying mechanism of the common causes of cerebral palsy:

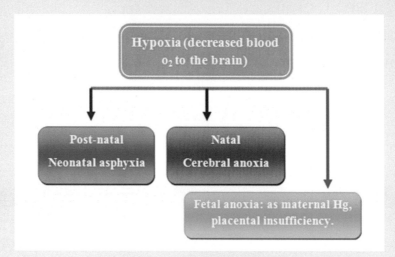

Fig (11): a-Hypoxia

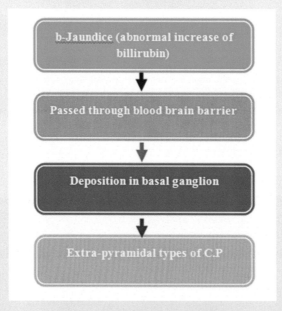

Fig (12): b-Jaundice

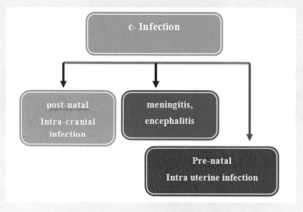

Fig (13): c- Infection

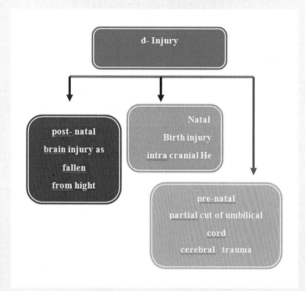

Fig (14): d- Injury

5-Underlying mechanism of types and forms of C.P

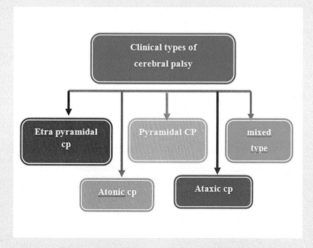

Fig (15): Types of cerebral palsy

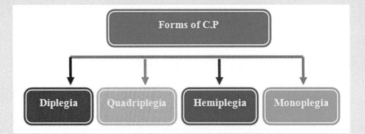

Fig (16): Forms of CP

6-Underlying mechanism of characteristics of different types of C.P:

Table: (7)

Pyramidal	Extra-pyramidal	atonic	ataxic	mixed
This is the most common clinical type which is characterized by: - Spasticity of the extremitiesExaggerated deep tendon reflex - Clonus - Positive babiniski sign - Abnormal persistence of neonatal reflexes - Scissoring of the lower limbs - Pseudo-bulbar palsy lead to	it is due to Bilirubin encephalopathy and is usually accompanied by deafness, basal ganglia is the most affected site it present by : - Rigidity - Chorea +or- athetosis (choreo –athetotic cp) - Dystonia - fluctuating hypertonia - involuntary movement - Wshape position - Dancing gait - Laxity of	sever 72ypotonia (floppy infant) - 72ypotonia 72 deep tendon reflex	Due to affection of cerebellum. it present by– 72ypotonia + hyporeflexia - un coordinated movement(intension tremor+gait ataxia) - nystagmus +staccato speech:- Hypotonia, some have hypertonia Poor co contraction- - Incoordination - Poorly coordinated postural reaction - difficult balance	a combination of 2 or more of the previous types
difficult swallowing, rolling of saliva, exaggerated gag reflex	ligament		and lurching gait,drunken gait,zigzag gait,wide base gait	

7-Underlying mechanism of physical problems of hemiplegia and spastic diaplegia:

Table: (8)

Hemiplegia	Spastic diaplegia
1- In prone : affected arm remain flexed under chest	1- Rolling : shoulder, pelvis and leg held stiffly, extended during rolling
2- Rolling : cannot roll on affected side	2- crawling : missing of the normal reciprocal creeping movement due to lack of flexion pattern at both legs
3- Late in sitting up and have balance problem	3- cannot make a long sitting
4- Standing : weight bearing on sound side use affected one for balance	4- pull up from supine to sitting leg extended stiffly, abduct with internal rotation and plantar flexion 5 - loss of balance of trunk in sitting
5- Walking : affected leg extended at knee drag it behind sound side shoulder retract, elbow flexed with fisted hand repeated falling due to weak equilibrium and protective reaction	6 - marked forward flexion of spine and shoulder girdle disturb sitting pattern
	7 - very weak protective reaction of the arms
	8 - W shape sitting is the only way for sitting for him
	9 - Cannot extend his hips fully ,to stand up pull himself up with his arms strength on to his toes then move his feet forward
	10 - walking holding on furniture with one foot flat other on toes

N.B Hypotonia can occur in cerebral palsy either **transient Hypotonia** (Transient hypotonia subsequently being spasticity if the child has colonus reflex or athetoid if there is tremors and involuntary movement or stereotyped movement, or ataxia if there is nystagmus .

- May have respiratory problem
- Dysphagia and drilling are common
- Developmental delay or **central Hypotonia** which continue with hypotnia as a result of pure lesion of area 4(pure pyramidal tract lesion)

8-Underlying mechanism of physical and neurological examination:

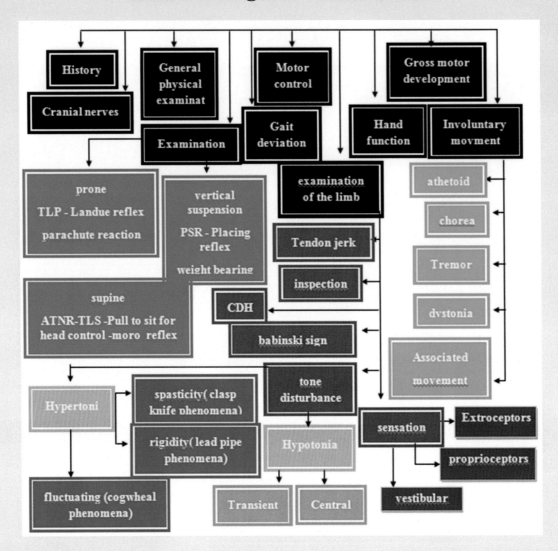

Fig (17): Physical and neurological examination of cerebral palsy

A-History taking :

1-Age in months some time in week.

2-Sex some disease related to sex(male or female)

3-Address some disease related to it(pollution)

4-Period in incubation(how long)

5-First cry(when)

6-Blue or yellow child(hypoxia or jaundice)

7-Mature or pre mature(full term or pre term)

8-Development and family information(familial disease and positive consanguinity)

B-Evaluation of motor control:

1-Postural reaction:

- Without righting reaction the patients will have difficulty in getting up from the floor, getting out of bed, sitting up and kneeling
- Without equilibrium reaction the patients will have difficulty in maintaining and recovering of balance in all positions and ADL activities
- Without protective reaction the patients suffering from repeated fallen, difficulty to bear weight on the affected side during normal ADL activities

Postural reactions components in evaluation: Table: (9)

Characteristics of reactions	Righting reaction	Equilibrium reaction	Protective reaction
1-Stimulus	By tilting	By disturbance	By forced movement
2-Response	Righting of head and thorax(axial part)	Upper side has equilibrium reaction, lower side has protective reaction and righting reaction on axial part	Step forward or backward or sideway to maintain balance
3-COG(center of gravity)	Within B.O.S	Within B.O.S	Outside B.O.S
4-Base of support(B.O.S)	Big	Small	Very small
5-End result of training(function outcome)	sitting	Standing and walking	Prevention of repeated fallen

2-Reflexes:

Spinal reflexes:

1-Flexor withdrawal reflex

2-Extensor thrust

3-Crossed extension 1

4-Crossed extension 2

Brain stem reflexes(tonic reflexes)

1-ATNR(Asymmetrical tonic neck reflex)

2-STNR 1(symmetrical tonic neck 1)

3-STNR2(symmetrical tonic neck2)

4-TLS(tonic labyrinthine supine)

5-TLP(tonic labyrinthine supine)

6-PSR(positive supporting reaction)

Mid brain level

1-Labyrnthine righting (with closed eyes) to right, to left anterior, posterior

2-Optical righting (with open eyes)

the same

3-Neck righting

4-Body righting acting on body

Cortical level (equilibrium reaction)

1-Supine

2-Prone

3-Quadriped

4-Sitting

5-kneeling

6-Dorsiflexion

7-Squating

- **Asymmetrical tonic neck reflex interfere with gross motor skills as rolling and fine motor skills as hand function, feeding, eye hand co ordinationas following:**

- Cannot bring an object to the mouth
- Cannot hold an object in both hands
- Cannot grasp an object in front of the body while looking at
- Cannot move both arms in midline

- **Symmetrical tonic neck reflex:** Interfere with all functional activities

- **Positive supporting reaction:** The patients will have difficulty in: Getting up from, sitting in a chair, walking down steps, maintain balance in standing, sitting, balance, weight shift, rolling

- **Grasp reflex:** The patients will have difficulty in all hand manipulative skills (grasping, reaching, eye hand co ordination) and interfere with parachute reaction, weight bearing.

- **Tonic labyrinthine supine, prone:** Interfere with pull to sit, rolling, prone on hand or hand support

-**Moro reflex:** interfere with rolling, eye hand co ordination, balance

C-General physical examination:
Anthropometric measures:
a-Weights
normal birth 2.5-3.5k
at 1 year= 9 kg
after 2nd year:
weight=age in year× 2+8
b- Length or height
normal birth length=50cm
at 1 year=75cm
after 4 year
length=age×5+80
c- Head circumference
at birth: 35cm
at6 months:43cm

at 1 year45cm

at 2 years 47cm

at 5 years 50cm

d- Fontanel's:

6 Fontanelles: 1anterior,1posterior,2 sphenoid and 2 mastoid

All are closed before 6 months except ant. Fontanel closed normally at 18 months

At birth become 3 finger bridth

At 6 months become 2 finger bridth

At 12 months become 1 finger bridth

At 18 months will be closed

D-Gross motor development

Gross motor (large muscle) **development** refers to improvement of skills and control of the large muscles of the legs, arms, back and shoulders which are used in walking, sitting, running, jumping, climbing, and riding a bike.

Gross motor skills occur in a typical sequence. However, these skills can only occur as the infant develops the balance, coordination and postural control, inhibit all primitive reflexes needed to move his body about in space

Pre-requisites for the development of head control:

Intact vestibular system

Intact eyes and optical pathways

Intact proprioceptors of neck region

Intact neck structures including joints, capsules, ligaments and muscles

Sequence of development of head control:

2 weeks	turning head to the side
1-2 months	raising head from prone
3-5 months	raising head from supine
5-7 months	raising head from side lying

Rolling

Pre requisites:

Development of head control(even partially)

Development of neck righting reaction

Development of the ability to support on forearms and hands

Sequences:

Turning start reflexly from supine to side lying	1-4months
Turning from prone to supine	4-5 months
Turning from supine to prone	5-7 months

By 7 months he can roll voluntary from prone to supine and from supine to prone

Sitting

Pre requisites:

The ability to raise the trunk against gravity

The ability to support on the upper limbs

Pivoting (trunk rotation)

Sequences:

4 weeks	sit with rounded back
4-5 months	can sit with support
6-7 months	sit with back support by chair
7-8 months	sit without support

Creeping

Four points mobility by both hands and knees on the floor

Pre requisites:

The ability to support on upper limbs and knees

The ability to do reciprocal movement of hands and legs

The ability to raise the trunk against gravity

Sequences: Age ranged; 8-10 months

Standing

Pre requisites:

Intact vestibular system

Emergence of postural reaction

Intact lower limbs musculo- skeletal system

Sequences:

Pull to stand	10 10.5months
Standing holding on	11-12months
Stand without assistance	13-15 months

Walking
Pre requisites:
- Intact vestibular system
- Well developed postural reaction
- Intact lower limbs musculo skeletal system

Sequences:

First step can walk with help	12 months
Independent walking	15-18 months

Walking up and down stairs:	2 years
Jumping:	2.5 years
Running:	3 years

Headcontrol
Is the first movement that a baby achieves, and is necessary to attain other movement skills such as sitting, crawling, and walking Head control: requires strength and coordination of the muscles which flex and extend the neck. A baby will develop head control in 3 major positions; prone, supine and in sitting

Rolling
Rolling from stomach to back
then from back to stomach
It is important for these infants to spend some time on their stomach, however, as many skills are developed when a child plays in this position

Sitting
The ability to maintain a sitting position requires a baby to have developed righting reaction responses in the forward, backward, and side to side directions.

If a baby has difficulty with maintaining balance, his righting reactions must be improved by training him in the sitting position.

- Transient sitting: using of hands support in front then in side for maintain sitting balance
- Complete sitting: alone

If a baby has muscle tightness in his legs, or weakness in his neck or trunk muscles sitting will be more difficult for the baby

Pull to stand and side walking

This sidestepping teaches the weight shift of infant which will need to take steps forward in walking

Standing

- Standing with support
- Standing with hold on
- Standing alone

Walking

- Closed environment
- Open environment

Running and jumping

E-Evaluation of hand functions (grasping-voluntary release-eye hand coordination-bilateral hand use-hand manipulative skills-reaching):

Fine motor (small muscle) **development** refers to use of the small muscles of the fingers and hands for activities such as grasping objects, holding, cutting, drawing, buttoning, or writing

<u>Graduations level of material used in Azzam reacquisition hand skill grading scale:</u>

1-Big object, rectangular shape, rough, heavy, ↑time, ↓speed, ↑accuracy, ↓numbers of trials

2-Big object, rectangular shape, rough, heavy, ↓time, ↑speed, ↓accuracy, ↑number of trials

3-Big object, square shape, rough, heavy, ↑time, ↓speed, ↑accuracy, ↓numbers of trials

4-Big object, square shape, rough, heavy, ↓time, ↑speed, ↓accuracy, ↑number of trials

5-Big object, rectangular, rough, light, ↑time, ↓speed, ↑accuracy, ↓numbers of trials

6-Big object, rectangular, rough, light, ↓time, ↑speed, ↓accuracy, ↑number of trials

7-Big object, rectangular, smooth, heavy, ↑time, ↓speed, ↑accuracy, ↓numbers of trials

8-Big object, rectangular, smooth, heavy, ↓time, ↑speed, ↓accuracy, ↑number of trials

9-Big object, circular, rough, heavy, ↑time, ↓speed, ↑accuracy, ↓numbers of trials

10-Big object, circular, rough, heavy, ↓time, ↑speed, ↓accuracy, ↑number of trials

11-Big object, rectangular, smooth, light, ↑time, ↓speed, ↑accuracy, ↓numbers of trials

12-Big object, rectangular, smooth, light, ↓time, ↑speed, ↓accuracy, ↑number of trials

13-Big object, circular, smooth, heavy, ↑time, ↓speed, ↑accuracy, ↓numbers of trials

14-Big object, circular, smooth, heavy, ↓time, ↑speed, ↓accuracy, ↑number of trials

15-Big object, circular, smooth, light, ↑time, ↓speed, ↑accuracy, ↓numbers of trials

16-Big object, circular, smooth, light, ↓time, ↑speed, ↓accuracy, ↑number of trials

17-Big object, rectangular, rough, light ↑time, ↓speed, ↑accuracy, ↓numbers of trials

18-Big object, rectangular, rough, light, ↓time, ↑speed, ↓accuracy, ↑number of trials

19-Big object, square, rough, light ↑time, ↓speed, ↑accuracy, ↓numbers of trials

20-Big object, square, rough, light, ↓time, ↑speed, ↓accuracy, ↑number of trials

21-Small object, rectangular, rough, heavy, ↑time, ↓speed, ↑accuracy, ↓numbers of trials

22-Small object, rectangular, rough, heavy, ↓time, ↑speed, ↓accuracy, ↑number of trials

23-Small object, square, rough, heavy, ↑time, ↓speed, ↑accuracy, ↓numbers of trials

24-Small object, square, rough, heavy, ↓time, ↑speed, ↓accuracy, ↑number of trials

25-Small object, circular, rough, heavy, ↑time, ↓speed, ↑accuracy, ↓numbers of trials

26-Small object, circular, rough, heavy, ↓time, ↑speed, ↓accuracy, ↑number of trials

27-Small object, rectangular, smooth, heavy, ↑time, ↓speed, ↑accuracy, ↓numbers of trials

28-Small object, rectangular, smooth, heavy, ↓time, ↑speed, ↓accuracy, ↑number of trials

29-Small object, rectangular, rough, light ↑time, ↓speed, ↑accuracy, ↓numbers of trials

30-Small object, rectangular, rough, light, ↓time, ↑speed, ↓accuracy, ↑number of trials

31-Small object, square, rough, light ↑time, ↓speed, ↑accuracy, ↓numbers of trials

32-Small object, square, rough, light, ↓time, ↑speed, ↓accuracy, ↑number of trials

33-Small object, rectangular, smooth, light, ↑time, ↓speed, ↑accuracy, ↓numbers of trials

34-Small object, rectangular, smooth, light, ↓time, ↑speed, ↓accuracy, ↑number of trials

35-Small object, square, smooth, light, ↑time, ↓speed, ↑accuracy, ↓numbers of trials

36-Small object, square, smooth, light, ↓time, ↑speed, ↓accuracy, ↑number of trials

37-Small object, circular, smooth, heavy, ↑time, ↓speed, ↑accuracy, ↓numbers of trials

38-Small object, circular, smooth, heavy, ↓time, ↑speed, ↓accuracy, ↑number of trials

39-Small object, circular, rough, light, ↑time, ↓speed, ↑accuracy, ↓numbers of trials

40-Small object, circular, rough, light, ↓time, ↑speed, ↓accuracy, ↑number of trials

41-Small object, circular, smooth, light ↑time, ↓speed, ↑accuracy, ↓numbers of trials

42-Small object, circular, smooth, light, ↓time, ↑speed, ↓accuracy, ↑number of trials

N.B, The time required to perform the level in normal from 180sec to 200 sec. We use the stop watch to measure the time performance the more decrease in time of performance indicate to improvement in gaining the skill

F- Gait deviations in pediatric: Table: (10)

Form of cerebral palsy	Type of gait disturbance	The cause of gait disturbance
Hemiplegic cerebral palsy	Circumduction or hip hiking gait	Spasticity of quadrates lumborum
	Toe gait	Tightness of hamstring and tendo-achilis muscles
	High steppege gait	Weakness or paralysis of anterior tibial group
Spastic diaplegia	Crouch gait	Mild spasticity of hip adductors
	Scissor gait	sever spasticity of hip adductors
Dyskinesia	Dancing gait	Released of flexor withdrawal reflex
Cerebellar ataxia	drunken, zigzage, limb gait	unilateral lesion of cerebellum
	wide base gait	bilateral lesion
	trunkal gait	tendency of trunk to fall backward lesion in vermis
	stamping gait	impaired of deep sensation

Sensory ataxia		
Myopathy	Lurching gait	Bilateral Weakness of gluteus maximums muscle
	Waddling gait	Bilateral Weakness of gluteus medius muscle
Poliomyelitis	Hand to knee gait	Weakness or paralysis of quadriceps
	Limping gait	Leg length discrepancy
Guillian baree syndrome	High steppege gait	Weakness or paralysis of anterior tibial group muscles
Juvenile rheumatoid arthritis	Antalgic gait	Due to pain
Muscle weakness	Trendlenburg gait	Unilateral weakness of gluteus medius
	Lurching gait	Bilateral weakness of both glueus maximus
	Waddling gait	Bilateral weakness of both glueus medius
	High steppege gait	Weakness or paralysis of anterior tibial group muscles
	Hand to knee gait	Weakness or paralysis of quadriceps

Underlying mechanism of cerebral palsy treatment:

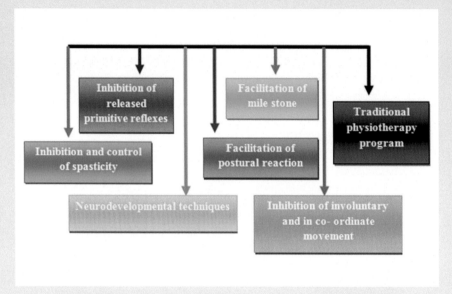

Fig (18): Treatment lines of cerebral palsy

Inhibition and control of spasticity:

Prolonged stretch to spastic muscle to gain relaxation via: At first quick stretch occur lead to stimulate gamma fibers lead to stimulate con-tractile part of intra-fusal muscle fiber lead to stimulate non contractile part which include stretch receptors sending afferent signals to PHC Then to AHC then to alpha motor neuron causing contraction of extra-fusal muscle fibers.

At second step just one contraction or repeated contraction occurred stimulate GTO sending 1b afferent to PHC then to 1b inter neuron which reverses the stimulated signals into inhibitory signals. Then inhibit AHC then inhibit alpha motor neuron then relaxate extra-fusal muscle fibers. Techniques used as prolonged stretch (positioning, night splint, reflex inhibiting pattern, Bobath technique)

In most cases the abnormal pattern is due to combined forces of shortening and spasticity of the involved muscles (long-standing uncontrolled spasticity results in shortening of the muscle fibers and muscle sheath).

So these combined pathological mechanism is in bad need for proper physiotherapy program (via eliminate hyperirritability of the spastic muscles) plus adjustable static and dynamic splint (decrease and release of muscle and sheath contracture, relaxation of spastic muscles, stimulate Proprioceptive and cutaneous receptors by creating a deep pressure effect on the skin, inhibitions of pathologic reflexes and create the support needed to stabilize the extremities). The decrease of spasticity and tightness also help in development of muscle balance.

Methods of inhibition and control of Spasticity:

1-Ice application:
- Prolonged application on spastic muscles with looking at hyperemia every minute to avoid burn will produce inhibition of gamma fiber.
- Brief application on anti-spastic muscle will produce firing of gamma fibers of anti-spastic muscle which produce reciprocal inhibition of spastic muscles.

2-Vestibular stimulation:
Static(in linear acceleration) or dynamic(in angular movement) vestibular stimulation stimulate crista ampularis and endolymph of semicircular canal stimulate vestibuo-cochlear nerve lead to stimulate the vestibule-spinal tract which modulate firing of alpha motor neuron leading to modulation of stretch reflexes of muscles leading to generalized relaxation of spasticity.

3-Balance training:
Balance contain three receptors(vision, vestibular system and proprioceptors) all these receptors are including in balance training we can isolate the vision by covering the eyes and isolate proprioceptors by standing on disturbed board so the concentration will be on vestibular stimulation. Vestibular system cannot be isolated it must included in balance training. Balance contain three components (righting reaction, equilibrium reaction and protective reaction)

Inhibition of spasticity occurred via vestibular stimulation, propricptive stimulation and facilitation of postural reaction components which leasd to sensory information lead to sensory motor integration and end by motor strategy which mean gaining of function after decreasing of spasticity.

4-Faradic stimulation:

electric-stimulation of anti-spastic muscles produce depolarization of the skin and muscle produce contraction of anti-spastic muscle which stimulate the reciprocal inhibition mechanism by contraction of ant-spastic muscle and relaxation of spastic one.

5-Vibration:

- Vibration by high frequency on anti-spatic muscle lead to stimulation of Ia afferent leading to muscle activation and reciprocally relax the spastic one via reciprocal inhibition mechanism.
- Vibration by low frequency on spastic muscle lead to inhibition of Ia afferent due to adaptation leading to relaxation of spastic muscle

6-Approximation:

Static (weight bearing) and dynamic (manual approximation and walking) approximation stimulate the static and dynamic proprioceptors which transferred to dorsal Colum tracts which localized by sensory area and smoothening by cerebellum and basal ganglion aiming for engramed to motor area and modulate the tone surrounding. Slow approximation used to inhibit spasticity.

7-Irradiation

Using resistance to strong muscle for firing of motor neuron pool of weak muscles.

8-Trigggering of mass flexion

Stimulate the flexion pattern in L.L produce inhibition of extensor spasticity via(clenching of toes, painful stimuli to sole of the foot,firm pressure to shaft of tibia and electric stimulation to anterior tibial group) produce mass flexion of LL leading to relaxation of extensor spasticity.

9-Positioning

- Quadruped position is recommended due to it has the following effects (prolonged stretch to flexors of upper limbs and extensors of lower limb-static approximation-inhibition of primitive reflexes –inhibition of released abnormal pattern). Produce reflex inhibiting pattern leading to relaxation of spastic muscles.

10-Prolonged stretch

Prolonged stretch to spastic muscle to gain relaxation via: At first quick stretch occur lead to stimulate gamma fibers lead to stimulate con-tactile part of intra-fusal muscle fiber lead to stimulate non contractile part which include stretch receptors sending afferent signals to PHC then to AHC then to alpha motor neuron causing contraction of extra-fusal muscle fibers. At second step just one contraction or repeated contraction occurred stimulate GTO sending 1b afferent to PHC then to 1b inter neuron which reverses the stimulated signals into inhibitory signals. Then inhibit AHC then inhibit alpha motor neuron then relaxate extra-fusal muscle fibers. Techniques used as prolonged stretch (positioning, night splint, reflex inhibiting pattern, Bobath technique)

11-Night splint

Produce prolonged stretch aiming for relaxation of spastic muscles and passive stretch for tight muscles

12-Casting

Produce prolonged stretch aiming for relaxation of spastic muscles and passive stretch for tight muscles

13-Biofeedback

Visual and auditory stimulation to anti-spastic muscles produce reciprocal inhibition of spastic muscles

14-Bobath technique

Depend on putting the spastic limb in (positioning, reflex inhibiting pattern, facilitation of postural reaction) using proximal and distal key point of control. Bobath technique leading to relaxation of spastic muscles via prolonged stretch

15-Topical anesthesia

- desensitization of the skin+ inhibition of gamma fiber of spastic muscles via spraying of anesthesia in one direction 3- 5 times then distribute it all over the spastic muscles cover it and leave for a minutes will produce relaxation.

16-Facilitate to anti-spastic muscle

Via tactile stimulation+ quick stretch +active contraction

Produce reciprocal inhibition to spastic muscles

17-Placing technique

Weight bearing to spastic limb on anti-spastic position produces prolonged stretch on spastic muscles and relaxation by putting upper limb in extension and lower in flexion and maintain position will produce relaxation.

18-Inverted head position

one method of vestibular stimulation(lateral and antero-posterior swinging from upside-down (static vestibular stimulation) and rotatory movement from upside down(dynamic vestibular stimulation) produce generalized relaxation via stimulation of vestibu-lospinal tracts which modulate alpha motor neuron and in sequence modulate stretch reflex of spastic muscles.

19- Hot packs

Stimulate arterial receptors leading to vasodilatation and increase of elasticity of spastic muscles leading to decrease tension of extroceptors on spastic muscles.

20-Graduated active ex. for anti- spastic muscles:

Starting with tapping followed by passive movement on anti-spastic muscles till the patient share in (active assisted) then active participation producing reciprocal inhibition to spastic muscles.

Inhibition of released primitive reflexes:

1-Grasp reflex

The inhibition of the reflex can be achieved by:

A-Hand weight bearing from quadruped and side sitting position.

B-Reflex inhibiting pattern for U.L from sitting position as thumb extension pattern as distal key point of control.

C-Encourage hand function as reaching and voluntary release

2-Asymmetrical tonic neck reflex
To inhibit this reflex:
A-positioning:
- Encourage the child to assume side lying position
- Quadruped position

B-Reflex inhibiting pattern:
From sitting position (on roll, on lap) apply the following pattern using **proximal key point of control:**
- All outward rotation.
- Horizontal abduction.
- Extension diagonal.
- Elevation.

C-Break- down the pattern of reflex.
When child in supine lying position, the head rotated to one side, the therapist adducts the arm on the face side and extend the arm on the occipital side.
D-Approximation
to the head and upper limb to normalize the muscle tone (slow, rhythmic).
E-Facilitation of postural reactions
F-Encourage hand function.

3-Positive supporting reaction
This reflex can be inhibited by:
A-Approximation: for L.L (slow, regular and rhythmic)
B-Positioning e.g.: quadruped, sitting on roll and squatting.
C- Reflex inhibiting pattern.
- Dorsiflexion of toes and ankle as distal key point of control
- Flexion, abduction and external rotation as proximal key point of control

D-Facilitation of dorsiflexion by
- Tapping in the anterior tibial group
- Painful stimulus to sole of the foot
- Pressure on the medial tibial plateau or medial malleolus

E-Facilitation of rolling and walking

Facilitation of delayed mile stone

1-Facilitation of head control:
A-From prone:
- On roll and make bilateral elevation of shoulder
- On wedge tapping on forehead, painful stimuli on nose,
- On wedge make scapular retraction with paraspinal stimulation
- On wedge raising to on limb sudden drop then raising both limbs sudden drop
- On ball bounce the ball
- On ball facilitation of righting and equilibrium reaction, protective reaction

B-Supine
- Pull to sit
- Pull to sit with painful stimuli on sternum
- Approximation must be slow in all cases
- Facilitation of postural reaction on ball

C-Sitting
- Approximation must be slow in all cases
- Bilateral extension diagonal
- Bilateral horizontal abduction
- Bilateral elevation without ward rotation

2-Facilitation of rolling:
A-Blanket and two therapists raise the blanket from one side to initiate rolling
B-Sponge mattress pressure on it from one side
C-Counter rotation
- Shoulder against pelvis
Pelvis against shoulder

Shoulder, pelvis against each other

3-Facilitation of sitting:

A-Facilitation of trunk control by approximation of trunk on sitting

B-From supine to side sitting on wedge

C-Sitting on adjustable chair and support lower limb and foot on wedge

D-Sitting on chair and table in front of him to support him and lower it gradually when occur improvement in trunk control

E-Righting, equilibrium and protective reaction onball

F-Sitting on corner

G-Counter poisoning reaching while sitting

H- Static sitting with arm supported without arm supported from cross sitting long sitting, ring sitting

4-Facilitation of standing:

A-From supine to stand

B-From prone to quadruped to kneeling to half kneeling to standing by holding him from pelvis

C-Approximation of lower limbs

D-Standing frame

E-Manual standing by locking knee

F-Equilibrium reaction from standing

G-Standing with disturbance with holding a stand bar

H-Step forward and back ward with disturbance

I-Standing on one leg with disturbance

J-Standing on balance board

K-Standing on corner and disturbance

L-Stoop and recovery from flexion trunk and return, from squatting to standing

5-Facilitation of walking:

1-Closed environment

Between parallel bars hold him from axilla at shoulder level then make reciprocal movement

Using obstacles while I hold him like walking

2-Open environment

Gait training while child completely independent

Walk on wedge then between rolls as obstacles

Walk in one line, side way, one leg pass the other leg in side walking

Traditional physiotherapy program

1-Training of pelvic stability and equal weight shift on both sides

2-Approximation technique for the upper and lower limbs

3-Training of active trunk extension for improving postural control and balance

4-Graduated active ex for trunk lower and upper limb muscles

5- Passive stretching ex. For tight muscles

6- Gait training ex.

F-Postural reaction training

Righting reactions can be trained in antero-posterior and lateral direction, oblique and other directions. Righting reaction training started by facilitation of rolling in different position. Sitting on an unstable surface moving arms or legs to shift center of gravity – Sitting on unstable surface in combination with traditional lifting exercises .When your vestibular system senses that your body is not erect, it triggers the righting reflex by stimulating the vestibular system which stimulate vestibule-spinal tract which modulate the gamma fibers lead to modulate stretch reflex lead to modulate abnormal co-contraction and posture sway in sitting leading to improvement of core stability and sitting balance. The first step for gaining righting reaction is the facilitation of rolling till the child participates by active rolling.

Once the child gain active rolling righting reaction is responded and sitting can be gained

The key for gaining standing balance is the equilibrium reaction training(via disturbance in different position with decrease of the BOS with maintaining on COG within base of support the functional end result of practice and repeated training are standing and walking).

The key for prevent repeated falling is protective reaction training by training of hopping reaction +parachute reaction in addition to equilibrium reaction(via forced movement which move the COG out side BOS make great disturbance the functional end result of practice and repeated training is prevent repeated falling.

Postural reactions components training: Table (11)

Characteristics of reactions	Righting reaction	Equilibrium reaction	Protective reaction
1-Stimulus	By tilting	By disturbance	By forced movement
2-Response	Righting of head and thorax(axial part)	Upper side has equilibrium reaction, lower side has protective reaction and righting reaction on axial part	Step forward or backward or sideway to maintain balance
3-COG(center of gravity)	Within B.O.S	Within B.O.S	Outside B.O.S
4-Base of support(B.O.S)	Big	Small	Very small
5-End result of training(function outcome)	sitting	Standing and walking	Prevention of repeated fallen

G-Inhibition of involuntary and in co-ordinated movement:

1- Frinkles co-ordinated ex:

1- Supine : hip and knee flexion and extension of each limb, foot flat on plinth .
2- Hip abduction and adduction of each limb with the foot flat, knee flexed: then with knee extended.

3- Hip and knee flexion and extension of each limb, heel lifted off plinth 4-Heel of one limb to opposite leg (toes, ankle, shin, patella) .

5- Heel of one limb to opposite knee, sliding down crest of tibia to ankle.

6- Hip and knee flexion and extension of both limbs, legs together.

7- Reciprocal movements of both limbs-flexion of one leg during extension of the other

8- Sitting: knee extension and flexion of each limb.

9- Sitting: hip abduction and adduction.

10- Sitting: alternate foot placing to a specified target.

11- Standing up and sitting down.

12- Standing: foot placing to a specified target

13- Standing: weight shifting.

14- Walking: sideways or forward to a specified count.

15- Walking: turning around to a specified count

16-Finger to finger training

17-Finger to nose training

18-Finger to physiotherapist finger training

N.B -All co ordinate ex. should begin with slow movement then more difficult by rapid movement

- All co ordinate ex. should begin with opened eyes then more difficult with closed eyes

2-Inhibition of involuntary movement

1-Positioning:

As quadruped position and cross sitting position which has several benefits for inhibition of involuntary movement:

- Proprioceptive training ⟶ ↑sensory awareness and stability
- Prevent of delaying of bone growth ⟶ ↑physical growth of bone ⟶ prevent osteoporosis
- ↑muscles pull on bone ⟶ maintain muscle power and stimulate reciprocal inhibition between agonist and antagonist
- inhibition to released abnormal pattern produced by released tonic reflexes
- inhibition to involuntary movement and spasticity via prolonged stretch

2-Weight bearing as placing technique and hand weight bearing on both hands
- placing techniques by putting child in reflex inhibiting pattern bearing on his hands and reverse spastic pattern in lower limb
- weight bearing on both hands with elevation of both legs gradually
then walking in his hands to facilitate reciprocal movement of both hands
3-Stabilization of both hands and both legs by both hands of physiotherapist
4-Jerky approximation may help in inhibition of involuntary movement
5-Balance training produce vestibular stimulation which produces generalized inhibition to involuntary movement
6-Splinting can help in inhibition by preventing excessive activity

H-Underlying mechanism and effects of neuro- developmental technique

- Spasticity is the main physical problem facing the rehabilitation prognosis due to loss of normal reciprocal inhibition mechanism which produces smooth movement without clumsiness.
- Released of abnormal movement pattern is the second great problem due to released of tonic pathological reflexes which interfere with mile stone and functional activity producing inhibition of postural reaction mechanism which is the bridge to reach motor development
- Muscle tone disturbance occurred after CNS lesion may be either hypertonia (clasp knife phenomena as in spasticity-lead pipe phenomena as in rigidity and fluctuating hypertonia as in dyskinesia) or hypotonia (transient hypotonia which may become ataxic form if it is associated with nystagmus or become spastic if it is associated with colonus or become dyskinitic if it is associated with involuntary movement-central hypotonia which occurred due to pure lesion of area 4).
- Abnormal movement pattern due to muscle tone disturbance and released abnormal pattern reinforce abnormal perception-cognition complex which lead to abnormal motor engram resulting in child disability
- underlying mechanism of Bobath technique depends on prolonged stretch mechanism (explained in chapter 1).

- Inhibition of abnormal muscle tone,suppress of released abnormal pattern, increase joints awareness by proprioceptive stimulation,facilitations of postural reactions and facilitate perception –cognition complex are the keys for acquisition and re-acquisition of lost or impaired motor skill respectively.
- Reflex inhibiting pattern, positioning, proprioceptive training, facilitation of postural reactions, apply of distal and proximal key point of control

- Early intervention of NDT enable the rehabilitation team to reach the minimal cerebral palsy recovery due to more organization of the child abilities and early learning of normal sensory-motor experiences allow for normal body image which is the key for normal movement pattern before abnormal patterns of movement have become established

Underlying mechanism of neurodevelopment technique:

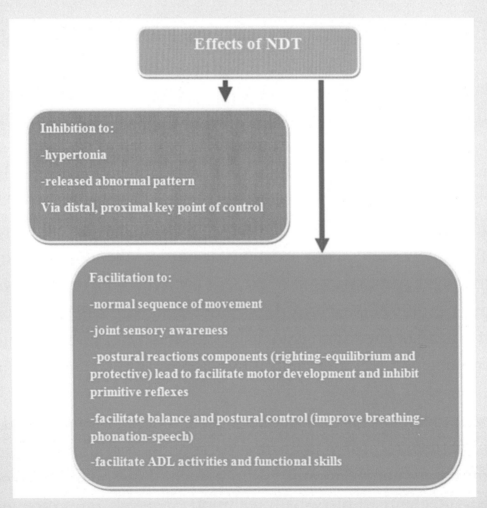

Fig (19): physiological effects of neurodevelopment technique

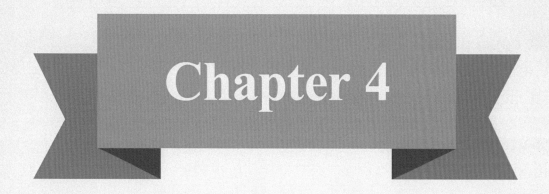

Chapter 4

Syndromes in pediatric rehabilitation

- Down syndrome
- Rett syndrome
- William syndrome
- Guillian Baree syndrome
- Arnold chiarri syndrome
- Horner syndrome
- Poliomyelitis and post-polio-syndrome

Factors affecting on growth and development:

1-Before conception:

a-Genetic factor: determination of the final height

b-Racial factors: white and black races are taller than yellow races

2-Intra-uterine factors:

- Nutritional state
- Maternal disease
- Maternal infection
- Maternal irradiation
- Maternal drug intake
- Maternal hypoxia

3-Post-natal factors

a. Age: maximum growth rate
   occur during infancy and early adolescent

b. Sex:
   until age of 11y growth rate of male>female
   from 11-14y growth rate of F>M and after 14 y growth rate of M>FS

C- Socio-economic factor

d- Psychological factor

e-Mal-nutrition lead to growth retardation

f-Endocrinal factors:

- Fetal period: growth under the effect of placental growth hormones
- Infancy and childhood under effect of growth hormone and thyroxin
- In adolescent under effect of sex hormones

Down syndrome

Underlying mechanisms of different types of down syndromes:

Types of human cells-

Somatic cells: All body cells except gonads. Divided by mitosis division giving 2 daughter cells has the same number of mother cell 46chr.

Germinal cells: Present only in gonads (ovary -testis) divided by meiosis producing 4cells

Two types of cell divisions

Mitosis: Goal is to produce two cells that are genetically identical to the parental cell.

Meiosis: Goal is to produce haploid gametes from adiploid parental cell. Gametes are genetically different from parent and each other.

Mitosis In mitosis the homologs do not pair up. Rather they behave independently. Each resultant cell receives one copy of each homolog.

MeiosisIn meiosis the products are haploid gametes so two divisions are necessary. Prior to the first division, the homologs pair up (synapse) and segregate from each other. In the second meiotic division sister chromatids segregate. Each cell receives a single chromatid from only one of the two homologs.

- Down syndrome is a chromosomal disorder that causes a lifelong Intellectual Disability, developmental delays and other problems
- Down syndrome varies in severity, so developmental problems range from moderate to serious
- Down syndrome is the most common chromosomal abnormality cause of learning disabilities in children
- Increased understanding of Down syndrome and early interventions make a big difference in the lives of both children and adults with Down syndrome
- Human cells normally contain 23 pairs of chromosomes—one chromosome in each pair comes from the father, the other from the mother.
- A chromosomaldisorder resulting from a partial or complete extra copy of chromosome 21.

Non-disjunction DS (94% of all cases): three complete copies in all cells.
Mosaicism DS (1-2% of cases): three copies in some but not all cells.
Translocation DS (3-4% of cases): partial copy of chromosome 21 attached to another chromosome.

Down syndrome: All of the cells contain extra chromosome to number21 chromosome

- Most of the time, down syndrome isn't inherited. It's caused by a mistake in cell division during the development of the egg, sperm or embryo
- Translocation Down syndrome is the only form of the disorder that can be passed from parent to child. However, only about 4% of children with Down syndrome have translocation. And only about half of these children inherited it from one of their parents

Risk factors include:

Some parents have a greater risk of having a baby with Down syndrome
- **Advancing maternal age.** A woman's chances of giving birth to a child with Down syndrome increase with age because older eggs have a greater risk of improper chromosome division. By age 35, a woman's risk of conceiving a child with Down syndrome is 1 in 400. By age 45, the risk is 1 in 35.
- **Having had one child with Down syndrome.** Typically, a woman who has one child with Down syndrome has about a 1% chance of having another child with Down syndrome
- **Being carriers of the genetic translocation for Down syndrome.** Both men and women can pass the genetic translocation for Down syndrome on to their children

Pathology of Down syndrome:

1-Non - disjunction DS (94%)
Related to maternal age

24chromosomes (ovum) × 23 Chromosome (sperm)

47chromosome in all of the cells

This form of Down syndrome is caused by abnormal cell division during the development of the sperm cell or the egg cell

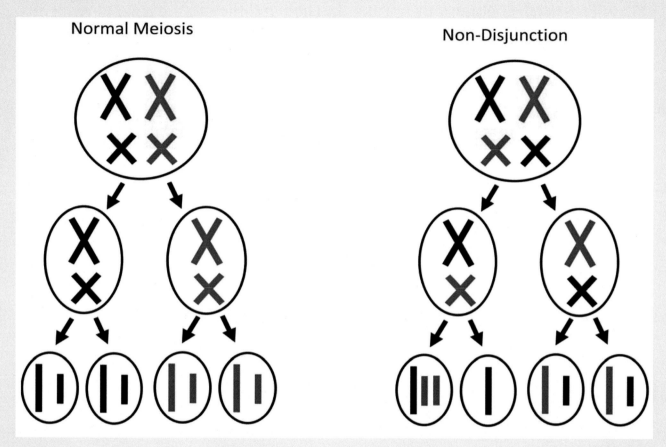

Fig (20): Non - disjunction DS

2- Translocation DS:

4% have the extra copy of chromosome 21 because of a translocation in which short arm of one chromosome exchanged with long arm of another one (14,21)

Down syndrome can also occur when part of chromosome 21 becomes attached (translocated) onto another chromosome, before or at conceptionChildren with translocation Down syndrome have the usual two copies of chromosome 21, but they also have additional material from chromosome 21 attached to the translocated Chromosome .This form of Down syndrome is uncommon

3- **1% have mosaicism DS:**

with normal and trisomy 21 cell lines (and usually have much milder features because of the presence of the normal cells); - occurs postzygotically (after fertilization)

Ovum (23) x sperm (23) lead to normal zygote (46ch.)

By division of zygote give 2 cells contain (46 ch.)

One of these cellscontinues its normal division and the other divide to two cells one of them contain 47 ch. And the other contains 45 ch. Which deadSo the child contain some normal cells (46ch) and abnormal cells (47ch)

Common sign and Symptoms:

- A distinct facial appearance:
- Flattened facial features
- Small head
- Short neck
- Protruding tongue
- Upward slanting eyes, unusual for the child's ethnic group
- Unusually shaped ears
- Poor muscle tone
- Broad, short hands with a single crease in the palm
- Relatively short fingers
- Excessive flexibility
- Infants with Down syndrome may be of average size, but typically they grow slowly and remain shorter than other children of similar age
- In general, developmental milestones, such as sitting and crawling, occur at about twice the age of children without impairment
- Children with Down syndrome also have some degree of Intellectual Disability, most often in the mild to moderate range
- 1 in 700 live births
>60% spontaneously aborted
20% stillborn

Multiple developmental and health effects including:
- Short stature, distinct facial features.
- Mild to moderate physical and cognitive impairment.

- Increased risk of problems involving heart, respiratory, digestive, hearing, vision, and/or thyroid glands.
- Facial appearance permits diagnosis
- Marked muscle hypotonia as baby
- Single palmar crease may be present
- Learning difficulty (IQ usually <50)
- Congenital heart malformations (40%)
- Many other associated features

Complications:
- Children with Down syndrome can have a variety of complications, some of which become more prominent as they get older, including:
- Heart defects. Approximately half the children with Down syndrome are born with some type of heart defect. These heart problems can be life-threatening and may require surgery in early infancy.
- Leukemia. Young children with Down syndrome are more likely to develop leukemia than are other children.
- Infectious diseases. Because of abnormalities in their immune systems, those with Down syndrome are much more susceptible to infectious diseases, such as pneumonia
- Dementia. Later in life, people with Down syndrome have a greatly increased risk of dementia. Signs and symptoms of dementia often appear before age 40 in people with Down syndrome. Those who have dementia also have a higher rate of seizures
- Sleep apnea. Because of soft tissue and skeletal alterations that lead to the obstruction of their airways, children with Down syndrome are at greater risk of obstructive sleep apnea
- Obesity. People with Down syndrome have a greater tendency to be obese than does the general population
- Other problems. Down syndrome may also be associated with other health conditions, including gastrointestinal blockage, thyroid problems, early menopause, seizures, hearing loss, premature aging, skeletal problems and poor vision

Life Expectancy:

Life spans have increased dramatically for people with Down syndrome
In 1929, a baby born with Down syndrome often didn't live to age 10
Today, someone with Down syndrome can expect to live to 50 and beyond, depending on the severity of his or her health problems

Evaluation of Down syndrome:

1-Muscle tone
2-Flexbility tests
3-Developmental age
4-Postural reaction
5-Reflexes
6-Gait
7-Hand function
8-Co-ordination
9-Functional muscletest and ROM tests
10-ADL activities
11-Learning skills
12-Social skills
13-Comminication skills
14-Cognitive skills

Physical problems of Down syndrome:

1-Hypotonia
2-Delaying mile stone
3-Laxity of ligament
4-Poor balance
5- Learning problems
6-Poor hand functions

Physiotherapy for Down syndrome:

1-Facilitation of Hypotonia)via facilitatory methods: approximation, taping followed by movement, quick stretch, rapping, electrical stimulation, vibration, pressure on bony prominence, clenching of toes, triggering of withdrawal reflex, weight bearing, ice,irradiation, jundracic maneuver, vestibular stimulation
2-Facilitation of mile stone
3-Functional strengthen ex.
4-Gait training
5-Orthoses
6-Hand function training
7-Facilitate learning abilities
8-Postural control:
- Postural reaction training
- Disturbance from different position
9-Co- ordination ex.
10-Graduated active ex.

Rett syndrome

Underlying mechanism of characteristics and physical problems in Rett syndrome:

Rett syndrome is a disorder of the nervous system that leads to developmental reversals, especially in the areas of motor, expressive language and hand use. Rett syndrome (RTT), originally termed cerebro-atrophic hyper-ammonemia, is a rare genetic postnatal neurological disorder of the greymatter of the brain[2] that almost exclusively affects females but has also been found in male patients. The clinical features include small hands and feet and a deceleration of the rate of head growth (including microcephaly in some). Repetitive stereotypedhand movements, such as wringing and/or repeatedly putting hands into the mouth, are also noted. People with Rett syndrome are prone to gastrointestinal disorders and up to 80% have seizures. They typically have no verbal skills, and about 50%

of affected individuals do not walk. Scoliosis, growth failure, and constipation are very common and can be problematic.

Genetically, Rett syndrome (RTT) is caused by mutations in the gene MECP2 located on the X chromosome. Rett syndrome is initially diagnosed by clinical observation, It has been argued that Rett syndrome is in fact a neuro-developmental condition as opposed to a neurodegenerative condition.

Causes:

Rett syndrome occurs almost always in girls. It may be misdiagnosed as autism or cerebral palsy. Studies have linked many Rett syndrome cases to a defect in a gene called methl-CpG-binding protein 2 (MeCP2). This gene is on the X chromosome. Females have two X chromosomes. Even when one chromosome has this defect, the other X chromosome is normal enough for the child to survive. Males born with this defective gene do not have a second X chromosome to make up for the problem. Therefore, the defect usually results in miscarriage, stillbirth, or very early death. The condition affects about 1 out of 10,000 children.

Signs of Rett syndrome those are similar to autism:

- Incontinence
- Screaming fits
- Inconsolable crying
- Breath holding, hyperventilation & air swallowing
- Avoidance of eye contact
- Lack of social/emotional reciprocity
- Markedly impaired use of nonverbal behaviors to regulate social interaction
- Loss of speech
- Sensory problems
- Signs of Rett syndrome that are also present in cerebral palsy (regression of the type seen in Rett syndrome would be unusual in cerebral palsy this confusion could rarely be made)
- Possible short stature, sometimes with unusual body proportions because of difficulty walking or malnutrition caused by difficulty swallowing
- Hypotonia in specific time
- Delayed or absent ability to walk

- Gait/movement difficulties
- Ataxia
- Microcephaly in some - abnormally small head, poor head growth
- Gastrointestinal problems
- Some forms of spasticity
- Chorea - spasmodic movements of hand or facial muscles
- Dystonia
- Bruxism – grinding of teeth

Signs may stabilize for many decades, particularly for interaction and cognitive function such as making choices. Asocial behavior may change to highly social behavior. Motor functions may slow as rigidity and dystonia appear. Seizures may be problematic, with a wide range of severity. Scoliosis occurs in most, and may require corrective surgery. Those who remain ambulatory tend to have less progression of scoliosis

Physical and occupational problems in Rett syndrome:

- Decreased breathing capacity
- Delaying motor development
- delaying of cranial nerve development leading to excessive saliva and drooling
- started by muscle weakness then may be transferred to spastic or dystonic or rigid muscle tone

- learning difficulties and decreased of intellectual abilities
- Scoliosis
- toe stiff gait
- Seizures
- delaying motor development
- sleep disturbance
- Loss of purposeful hand movements(delayed hand functions skills as grasping,eye hand co ordination,voluntary release,hand manipulative release, bilateral hand use and reaching) for example, the grasp used to pick up small objects is

replaced by repetitive hand motions like hand wringing or constant placement of hands in mouth
- delayed social and communication skills
- peripheral poor circulation
- delayed in speech development

How is Rett Syndrome Diagnosed?

A diagnosis of Rett syndrome is based on a girl's pattern of symptoms and behavior. The diagnosis can be made on these observations alone. Discussions between a doctor and a girl's parents will help determine important details, such as when symptoms started.

Genetic testing can help confirm the diagnosis in 80% of girls with suspected Rett syndrome. It's possible that genetic testing can help predict severity.

<u>Physical therapy for Rett syndrome:</u>

1-Facilitation of delayed mile stone (facilitate sitting, standing and walking)
2-Hand functions training (grasping, voluntary release, eye hand co ordination, hand manipulative skills, bilateral hand use and reaching)
3-Balance training(righting, equilibrium and protective reaction training)
- Disturbance from sitting, quadruped, kneeling, half kneeling and standing
4-Methods control muscle tone disturbance either in hypotonic stage or hypertonic(spastic or rigid or dystonic muscle tone)
5-ADL training
- Help with feeding and diapering(feeding training) OT's provide adaptive devices such as cuffs and loops (to help the individual hold their utensils), large handled utensils that are easier to grasp, and cups with lids to assist with eating and address proper nutrition. In general, all of these therapeutic methods are aimed at improving the quality of the swallowing response and general eating performance
- Signals such as opening their mouth in preparation for food, rejecting unwanted foods, and spending an increased amount of time watching their helpers,

indicates that guided feeding therapy can increase engagement in eating in some cases
- Methods to treat constipation (toilet training)
- dressing and undressing training
- One way OTs address this problem is by educating and encouraging caregivers to practice guided feeding. Guided feeding involves having the individual with RTT grasp the spoon and having the caregiver's hand over top of the child's in order to guide the movement of the individual to eat. The purpose of this therapy is to encourage involvement in this important self-care activity,

6-Weight bearing ex. to maintain muscle power, Proprioceptive training passive stretching to muscles and modulate of muscle tone disturbance)

7-Treatment of scoliosis by determine the convex side(the side of the hump) and concave side

Stretching ex for the concave side and graduated active ex, for the convex side

8-Increasing the patient's communication and cognitive skills and especially with augmentative communication strategies

9-Parental counseling

10-Occupationaltherapy as sensory integration therapy (facilitate extroceptors, proprioceptors and vestibular sensation) and facilitate learning abilities

11-Speech therapy for improving the languge and speech disorder

12-Hand splints place the hand in a more functional position and prevent repetitive motion; this leads to better finger and spoon-feeding skills

13-Active participation can be encouraged through the use of elbow splints, which decrease the repetitive stereotyped arm movement's characteristic of Rett. As a result, socialization and interaction with the environment during eating may increase

Prognosis
- An infant with Rett syndrome usually has normal development for the first 6 - 18 months. Symptoms range from mild to severe.
- The disease slowly gets worse until the teenage years. Then, symptoms may improve. For example, seizures or breathing problems tend to lessen in late adolescence.

- Developmental regression or delays vary. Usually, a child with Rett syndrome sits up properly but may not crawl. For those who do crawl, many do so by scooting on their tummy without using their hands.
- Similarly, some children walk independently within the normal age range, while others are delayed, don't learn to walk independently at all, or don't learn to walk until late childhood or early adolescence. For those children who do learn to walk at the normal time, some keep that ability for their lifetime, while other children lose the skill.
- Life expectancies are not well studied, although survival at least until the mid-20s is likely. The average life expectancy of a girl with Rett syndrome may be mid-40s. Death is often related to seizure, aspiration pneumonia, malnutrition, and accidents.

William's syndrome

(Opposite of autism)

Underlying mechanism of characteristics and physical problems in William syndrome:

William's syndrome is a developmental disorder that causes multiple developmental problems. Characterized by growth delays before and after birth (prenatal and postnatal growth retardation), This condition is characterized by mild to moderate intellectual disability or learning problems, unique personality characteristics, distinctive facial features, gross and fine motor delay and heart and blood vessel (cardiovascular) problems.

William's syndrome is a rare genetic disorder that affects a child's growth, physical appearance, and cognitive development. People who have William's syndrome are missing genetic material from chromosome 7, including the gene elastin. This gene's protein product gives blood vessels the stretchiness and strength required to withstand a lifetime of use. The elastin protein is made only during embryonic development and childhood, when blood vessels are formed. Because they lack the elastin protein, people with Williams Syndrome have disorders of the circulatory system and heart.

Also known as Williams–Beuren syndrome (WBS), is a rare neurodevelopmental disorder characterized by: a distinctive, "elfin" facial appearance, along with a low nasal bridge; an unusually cheerful demeanor and ease with strangers; developmental delay coupled with strong language skills; and cardiovascular problems.

<u>Pathology of William syndrome:</u>

It is caused by a deletion of about 26 genes from the long arm of chromosome number7. It occurs in 1 in 7,500 to 1 in 20,000 births. The syndrome was first identified in 1961 by New Zealander J.C.P. Williams A deletion is caused by a break in the DNA molecule that makes up a chromosome. In most cases, the chromosome break occurs while the sperm or egg cell (the male or female gamete) is developing. When this gamete is fertilized, the child will develop Williams's syndrome. The parent, however, does not have the break in any other cells and does not have the syndrome. In fact, the break is usually such a rare event that it is very unlikely to happen again if the parent has another child.

It is possible for a child to inherit a broken chromosome from a parent who has the disorder. But this is rare because most people with Williams's syndrome do not have children.

Deletions that happen during egg and sperm formation are caused by unequal recombination. Recombination normally occurs between pairs of chromosomes during meiosis. If the pairs of chromosomes don't line up correctly, or if the chromosome breaks aren't repaired properly, the structure of the chromosome can be altered. Unequal recombination occurs more often than usual at this location on chromosome 7, likely due to some highly repetitive DNA sequence that flanks the commonly deleted region

Physical and occupational therapy problems:

1-Delaying in gross motor development:

Williams's syndrome is also marked by a delay in development of motor skills. Infants with Williams develop the ability to lift their heads and sit without support months later than typically developing children. These delays continue into childhood, where patients with Williams's syndrome are delayed in learning to walk. In young children, the observed motor delay is around five to six months, though some research suggests that children with Williams's syndrome have a delay in development that becomes more extreme with age.

2-Delaying in fine motor skills and co ordination:

Children with motor delays as a result of Williams's syndrome are particularly behind in development of coordination, fine motor skills such as writing and drawing, response time, and strength and dexterity of the arms. Impaired motor ability persists (and possibly worsens) as children with Williams's syndrome reach adolescence.

3-Delaying in language abilities:

Developmental delays are present in most cases of Williams's syndrome, and include delay of language abilities and delayed motor skill development. Individuals with Williams's syndrome develop language abilities quite late relative to other children, with the child's first word often occurring as late as three years of age. Language abilities are often observed to be deficient until adolescence

4-Hypotonia then developing hypertonia with age:

As individuals with Williams's syndrome age, they frequently develop joint limitations and hypertonia, or abnormally increased muscle tone

5-Other general problems:

The most common problems of Williams's syndrome are heart defects, and unusual facial features. Other problems include failure to gain weight appropriately in infancy (failure to thrive), and low muscle tone. Individuals with Williams's syndrome tend to have widely spaced teeth, a long philtrum, and a flattened nasal bridge.

Most individuals with Williams's syndrome are highly verbal relative to their IQ, and are overly sociable, having what has been described as a "cocktail party" type personality. Individuals with WS hyper focus on the eyes of others in social engagements.

It is in some respect the opposite of autism; individuals with WS are more sociable than those with autism, but those with WS have impairment in cognitive function as it relates to visuospatial functioning. Because of the multiple genes that are missing in people with Williams's syndrome, there are many effects on the brain, including abnormalities in the cerebellum, right parietal cortex, and left frontal cortical regions. This pattern is consistent with the visual-spatial disabilities and problems with behavioral timing often seen in Williams's syndrome.

Frontal-cerebellar pathways, involved in behavioral timing, are often abnormally developed in individuals with Williams's syndrome, which may be related to their deficits in coordination and execution of fine motor tasks such as drawing and writing. In addition, people with Williams's syndrome often exhibit gross motor difficulties, including trouble walking down stairs, as well as overactive motor reflexes (hyperreflexia) and hyperactive, involuntary movement of the eyes (nystagmus).

Williams syndrome are often able to visually identify and recognize whole objects, and refer to them by name, but struggle with visuospatial construction (seeing an object as being composed of many smaller parts, and recreating it) and orienting themselves in space.
Diagnosis of Williams's syndrome begins with recognition of physical symptoms and markers, which is followed by a confirmatory genetic test.

Treatment of William's syndrome:

1-Facilitation of delayed mile stone
2-Hand functions training (grasping, voluntary release, eye hand co ordination, bilateral hand use, hand manipulative skills and reaching)
3-Tone abnormality control (inhibitory techniques for hypertonia and facilitatory techniques for hypotonic period)

4-Balance training program (righting, equilibrium and protective reactions)

5-Proprioceptive training (static and dynamic approximation)

6-Weight bearing ex

7-Gait training

8-ADL training

9-Occupational therapy treatment (improve learning disabilities, hand functions, ADL and sensory motor integration)

10-Speech and language therapy

11-Improve social and communicating skills

Guillain-Barrè Syndrome

Underlying mechanism of characteristics and physical problems in Guillain-Barrè Syndrome:

Guillain-Barrè syndrome is a rare disorder in which body's immune system attacks nerves. Weakness and tingling in your extremities are usually the first symptoms.

Guillain-Barré syndrome (GBS) is a disorder in which the body's immune system attacks part of the peripheral nervous system. The first symptoms of this disorder include varying degrees of weakness or tingling sensations in the legs. In many instances the symmetrical weakness and abnormal sensations spread to the arms and upper body

These sensations can quickly spread, eventually paralyzing your whole body. In its most severe form Guillain-Barre syndrome is a medical emergency. Most people with the condition must be hospitalized to receive treatment.

The exact cause of Guillain-Barre syndrome is unknown. But it is often preceded by an infectious illness such as a respiratory infection or the stomach flu.

Guillain-Barré syndrome can affect anybody. It can strike at any age and both sexes are equally prone to the disorder. The syndrome is rare, however, afflicting only about one person in 100,000. Usually Guillain-Barré occurs a few days or weeks after the patient has had symptoms of a respiratory or gastrointestinal viral infection.

<u>Pathology:</u>

The nerve dysfunction in Guillain–Barré syndrome is caused by an immune attack on the nerve cells of the peripheral nervous system and their support structures. The nerve cells have their body (the soma) in the spinal cord and a long projection (the axon) that carries electrical nerve impulses to the neuromuscular junction where the impulse is transferred to the muscle. Axons are wrapped in a sheath of Schwann cells that contain myelin. Between Schwann cells are gaps (nodes of Ranvier) where the axon is exposed. Different types of Guillain–Barré syndrome feature different types of immune attack.

The demyelinating variant features damage to the myelin sheath by white blood cells (T lymphocytes and macrophages); this process is preceded by activation of a group of blood proteins known as complement. In contrast, the axonal variant is mediated by IgG antibodies and complement against the cell membrane covering the axon without direct lymphocyte involvement.
The body's immune system begins to attack the body itself, causing what is known as an autoimmune disease. Usually the cells of the immune system attack only foreign material and invading organisms. In Guillain-Barré syndrome, however, the immune system starts to destroy the myelin sheath that surrounds the axons of many peripheral nerves, or even the axons themselves (axons are long, thin extensions of the nerve cells; they carry nerve signals). The myelin sheath surrounding the axon speeds up the transmission of nerve signals and allows the transmission of signals over long distances.

The peripheral nerves' myelin sheaths are injured or degraded, the nerves cannot transmit signals efficiently. That is why the muscles begin to lose their ability to respond to the brain's commands, commands that must be carried through the nerve network. The brain also receives fewer sensory signals from the rest of the body, resulting in an inability to feel textures, heat, pain, and other sensations. Alternately, the brain may receive inappropriate signals that result in tingling, "crawling-skin," or painful sensations. Because the signals to and from the arms and legs must travel the longest distances they are most vulnerable to interruption. Therefore, muscle weakness and tingling sensations usually first appear in the hands and feet and progress upwards.

When Guillain-Barré is preceded by a viral or bacterial infection, it is possible that the virus has changed the nature of cells in the nervous system so that the immune system treats them as foreign cells. It is also possible that the virus makes the immune system itself less discriminating about what cells it recognizes as its own, allowing some of the immune cells, such as certain kinds of lymphocytes and macrophages, to attack the myelin. Sensitized T lymphocytes cooperate with B lymphocytes to produce antibodies against components of the myelin sheath and may contribute to destruction of the myelin. In two forms of GBS, axons are attacked by antibodies against the bacteria which react with proteins of the peripheral nerves .This autoimmune disease is caused by the body's immune system mistakenly attacking the peripheral nerves and damaging their myelin insulation. Sometimes this immune dysfunction is triggered by an infection. The diagnosis is usually made based on the signs and symptoms, through the exclusion of alternative causes, and supported by tests such as nerve conduction studies and examination of the cerebrospinal fluid.

Clinical subtypes of Guillian Barree syndrome: Table: (12)

Type	Symptoms	Nerve conduction studies	Antiganglioside antibodies
Acute inflammatory demyelinating polyneuropathy (AIDP)	Sensory symptoms and muscle weakness, often with cranial nerve weakness and autonomic involvement	Demyelinating polyneuropathy	No clear association
Acute motor	Isolated muscle	Axonal	GM1a/b, GD1a &

axonal neuropathy (AMAN)	weakness without sensory symptoms in less than 10%; cranial nerve involvement uncommon	polyneuropathy, normal sensory action potential	GalNac-GD1a
Acute motor and sensory axonal neuropathy (AMSAN)	Severe muscle weakness similar to AMAN but with sensory loss	Axonal polyneuropathy, reduced or absent sensory action potential	GM1, GD1a
Pharyngeal-cervical-brachial variant	Weakness particularly of the throat muscles, face, neck and shoulder muscles	Generally normal, sometimes axonal neuropathy in arms	Mostly GT1a, occasionally GQ1b, rarely GD1a

Symptoms of Guillain-Barrè syndrome:

The symptoms of Guillain-Barrè syndrome include:
- Progressive muscle weakness and paralysis affecting both sides of the body
- Jerky, uncoordinated movements
- Muscle aches, pains or cramps
- Odd sensations such as vibrations, buzzing or 'crawling' under the skin
- Blurred vision
- Dizziness
- Breathing problems.
- Numbness, tingling and pain in hands and feet and sometimes around the mouth and lips.
- Trouble speaking, chewing, and swallowing.
- In ability to move eyes.
- Back pain.
- Co-ordination problems and unsteadiness (may be unable to walk unaided)

- Symptoms usually start with numbness or tingling in the fingers and toes. Over several days, muscle weakness in the legs and arms develops. After about 4 weeks, most people begin to get better.
Recovery may take six months to two years or more.

Physical problems in Guillain-Barrè syndrome:

- In ability to walk unaided – for example, needing a wheelchair
- sensory ataxia (loss ofdeep) sensation that may cause a lack of co-ordination
- Loss of balance
- Muscle weakness in The muscles of the neck may also be affected, and about half experience involvement of the cranial nerves, which supply the head and face; this may lead to weakness of the muscles of the face, swallowing difficulties and sometimes weakness of the eye muscles, arms and legs (flaccid paraplegia)
- Problems with extro-ceptive sensationas touch often felt as a burning or tingling sensation
- Persistent fatigue (extreme tiredness).
- Hypotonia and hyporeflexia
- Tightness of tendoachilis and wrist muscles
- High steppege gait
- Hand function disturbance

Treatment of Guillian Barree syndrome:

1-Fcilitatory techniques to the paralyzed muscles(as faradic stimulation to ant-tibial group and wrist extensors)
2-Graduated active ex. to the weak muscles
3-Balance training program including righting, equilibrium, protective reaction
4-Mild, gentle and decent passive stretch to tight muscles
5-Splinting
- Night ankle foot splint to prevent and decrease tightness
- Dynamic ankle foot orthoses for improving gait pattern
6-Gait training (closed and open environment)
7-Facilitahion of hand function skills

8-Facilitation of ADL skills

9-Weight bearing ex.

10-Proprioceptive training via static and dynamic approximation

11- Speech therapy is aimed at promoting speech and safe swallowing skills for patients who have significant oropharyngeal weakness with resultant dysphagia and dysarthria.

Arnold chiarri syndrome

Underlying mechanism of characteristics and different types of Arnold chiarri Syndrome:

Chiari malformations (CMs) are structural defects in the cerebellum, the part of the brain that controls balance. Normally the cerebellum and parts of the brain stem sit in an indented space at the lower rear of the skull, above the foramen magnum (a funnel-like opening to the spinal canal). When part of the cerebellum is located below the foramen magnum, it is called a Chiari malformation.

CMs may develop when the bony space is smaller than normal, causing the cerebellum and brain stem to be pushed downward into the foramen magnum and into the upper spinal canal. The resulting pressure on the cerebellum and brain stem may affect functions controlled by these areas and block the flow of cerebrospinal fluid (CSF)— the clear liquid that surrounds and cushions the brain and spinal cord—to and from the brain.

Types of Chiari Malformations:

CMs are classified by the severity of the disorder and the parts of the brain that protrude into the spinal canal.

Type I:

Involves the extension of the cerebellar tonsils (the lower part of the cerebellum) into the foramen magnum, without involving the brain stem. Normally, only the spinal cord passes through this opening. Type I—which may not cause symptoms—is the most common form of CM and is usually first noticed in adolescence or adulthood, often by accident during an examination for another condition. Type I is the only type of CM that can be acquired.

Type II:

Also called classic CM, involves the extension of both cerebellar and brain stem tissue into the foramen magnum. Also, the cerebellar vermis (the nerve tissue that connects the two halves of the cerebellum) may be only partially complete or absent. Type II is usually accompanied by a myelomeningocelea form of spina bifida that occurs when the spinal canal and backbone do not close before birth, causing the spinal cord and its protective membrane to protrude through a sac-like opening in the back. A myelomeningocele usually results in partial or complete paralysis of the area below the spinal opening. The term Arnold-Chiari malformation (named after two pioneering researchers) is specific to Type II malformations.

Type III:

Is the most serious form of CM. The cerebellum and brain stem protrude, or herniate, through the foramen magnum and into the spinal cord. Part of the brain's fourth ventricle, a cavity that connects with the upper parts of the brain and circulates CSF, may also protrude through the hole and into the spinal cord. In rare instances, the herniated cerebellar tissue can enter an occipital encephalocele, a pouch-like structure that protrudes out of the back of the head or the neck and contains brain matter. The covering of the brain or spinal cord can also protrude through an abnormal opening in the back or skull. Type III causes severe neurological defects.

Type IV:

Involves an incomplete or underdeveloped cerebellum—a condition known as cerebellar hypoplasia. In this rare form of CM, the cerebellar tonsils are located in a normal position but parts of the cerebellum are missing, and portions of the skull and spinal cord may be visible. Another form of the disorder, under debate by some scientists, is Type 0, in which there is no protrusion of the cerebellum through the foramen magnum but headache and other symptoms of CM are present.

Other conditions associated with Chiarri malformations
Individuals who have a CM often have these related conditions:
- Hydrocephalus is an excessive buildup of CSF in the brain. A CM can block the normal flow of this fluid, resulting in pressure within the head that can cause mental defects and/or an enlarged or misshapen skull. Severe hydrocephalus, if left untreated, can be fatal. The disorder can occur with any type of CM, but is most commonly associated with Type II.
- Spina bifida is the incomplete development of the spinal cord and/or its protective covering. The bones around the spinal cord don't form properly, leaving part of the cord exposed and resulting in partial or complete paralysis. Individuals with Type II CM usually have a myelomeningocele, a form of spina bifida in which the bones in the back and lower spine don't form properly and extend out of the back in a sac-like opening.

- Syringomyelia, or hydromyelia, is a disorder in which a CSF-filled tubular cyst, or syrinx, forms within the spinal cord's central canal. The growing syrinx destroys the center of the spinal cord, resulting in pain, weakness, and stiffness in the back, shoulders, arms, or legs. Other symptoms may include headaches and a loss of the ability to feel extremes of hot or cold, especially in the hands. Some individuals also have severe arm and neck pain.

- CMs may also be associated with certain hereditary syndromes that affect neurological and skeletal abnormalities, other disorders that affect bone formation and growth, fusion of segments of the bones in the neck, and extra folds in the brain.

<u>Causes of Chiarri Malformations:</u>

- Chiarri malformations are usually caused by structural defects in the brain and spinal cord. These defects develop during fetal development.

- Due to genetic mutations or a maternal diet that lacked certain nutrients, the indented bony space at the base of the skull is abnormally small. As a result, pressure is placed on the cerebellum. This blocks the flow of the cerebrospinal fluid. That's the fluid that surrounds and protects the brain and spinal cord.

- CM has several different causes. It can be caused by structural defects in the brain and spinal cord that occur during fetal development, whether caused by genetic mutations or lack of proper vitamins or nutrients in the maternal diet. This is called primary or congenital CM. It can also be caused later in life if spinal fluid is drained excessively from the lumbar or thoracic areas of the spine either due to injury, exposure to harmful substances, or infection. This is called acquired or secondary CM. Primary CM is much more common than secondary CM.

Treatment:

- Surgery is the only treatment available to correct functional disturbances or halt the progression of damage to the central nervous system. Most individuals who have surgery see a reduction in their symptoms and/or prolonged periods of relative stability. More than one surgery may be needed to treat the condition.

Horner syndrome

Underlying mechanism of characteristics in Horner Syndrome:

A combinationof symptoms that arises when a group of nerves known as the sympathetic trunk is damaged. The signs and symptoms occur on the same side as the lesion of the sympathetic trunk. It is characterized by miosis (a constricted pupil), ptosis (a weak, droopy eyelid), apparent anhidrosis (decreased sweating), with or without enophthalmus (inset eyeball).

Horner syndrome (Horner's syndrome) results from an interruption of the sympathetic nerve supply to the eye and is characterized by the classic triad of miosis (ie, constricted pupil), partial ptosis, and loss of hemifacial sweating (ie, anhidrosis).

Causes of Horner syndrome include the following:

- Lesion of the primary neuron
- Brainstem stroke or tumor or syrinx of the preganglionic neuron – In one study, 33% of patients with brainstem lesions demonstrated Horner syndrome
- Trauma to the brachial plexus (klumks paralysis)
- Tumors (eg, Pancoast) or infection of the lung apex
- Lesion of the postganglionic neuron
- Dissecting carotid aneurysm

Signs and symptoms:

Signs that are found in patients on the affected side of the face include
- Partial ptosis
- Upside-down ptosis (slight elevation of the lower lid)
- Anhidrosis
- Miosis
- Pseudoenophthalmos (the impression that the eye is sunk caused by a narrow palpebral aperture)
- Papillary dilation lag
- Loss of ciliospinal reflex
- Bloodshot conjunctiva, depending on the site of lesion.
- Unilateral straight hair (in congenital Horner's syndrome)
- Heterochromia iridum (in congenital Horner's syndrome)

The most common causes in young children are birth trauma (klumpks paralysis) and a type of cancer called neuroblastoma.

Poliomyelitis and post-polio –syndrome

Underlying mechanism of characteristics and physical problems in poliomyelitis:

Definition:
It is an acute viral infection localize in motor neurons of the CNS specially spinal cord and brain stem causing LMNL without sensory loos

Recovery stage:
From 2 weeks to 2 years
- There is subsidance of odema period of neural plasticity (axonal sprouting)
- After 2 years recovery cannot occur due to no formation of new motor end plate axons is parallel to muscles

Chronic stage:
(After 3 years)

Pathology:

- From oral fecal route to pharynx to intestine to AHC
- Viral multiplication play a major role in neural damage

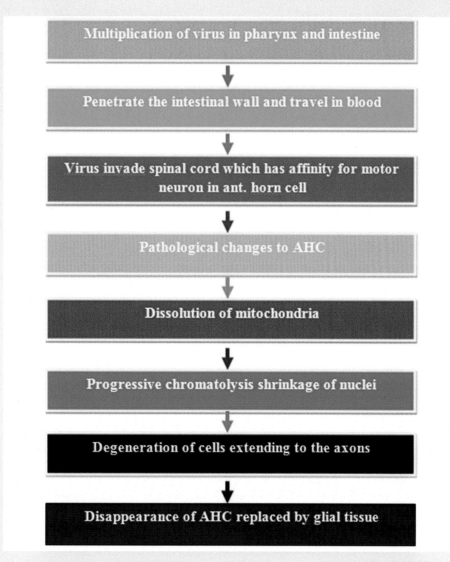

Fig (21): Underlying mechanism of poliomyelitis

Complications on musculoskeletal system:

1- Muscles

- Paralyzed muscles atrophied and replaced by C.T lead to shortening of muscle and tendon

2- Joints and bones

- Shortening in length and dislocated joints

3- Skin and subcutaneous tissues stasis and edematous of limbs

4- Respiratory system lung infection due to paralysis of diaphragm and intercostal muscles

Common deformities in polio

1- Hip joint: flexion abduction external rotation

2- knee joint: flexion deformity, genu recurvatum

3- Ankle joint: equinus, varus, valgus, pes cavus

Evaluation

1- History of vaccination

a- Salk: killed virus given by injection

b- Sabin: attenuated virus given orally

2- Informal evaluation (position of the limb, leg length discrepancy and deformities)

3- ROM

4- Long and round measurment

5- Postural assessment

6- Gait analysis

Treatment

1- Acute stage: positioning, hot packs, massage, passive ROM

2- Recovery and chronic stage

- Heat application

- Massage

- Stretching to tight muscles

- Graduated active ex

- Electrical stimulation

- TVR

- Biofeedback

- Hydrotherapy

- Splint and brace

Post-polio-syndrome

Post-polio syndrome refers to a cluster of potentially disabling signs and symptoms that appear decades an average of 30 to 40 years after the initial polio illness.

Post-polio syndrome (PPS) is a condition that affects polio survivors years after recovery from an initial acute attack of the poliomyelitis virus. Post-polio syndrome is rarely life-threatening, but the symptoms can significantly interfere with an individual's ability to function independently. Respiratory muscle weakness, for instance, can result in trouble with proper breathing, affecting daytime functions and sleep. Weakness in swallowing muscles can result in aspiration of food and liquids into the lungs and lead to pneumonia.

Most often, polio survivors start to experience gradual new weakening in muscles that were previously affected by the polio infection. The most common symptoms include slowly progressive muscle weakness, fatigue (both generalized and muscular), and a gradual decrease in the size of muscles (muscle atrophy). Pain from joint degeneration and increasing skeletal deformities such as scoliosis (curvature of the spine) is common and may precede the weakness and muscle atrophy. Some individuals experience only minor symptoms while others develop visible muscle weakness and atrophy.

Underlying mechanism of post-polio syndrome:

1-Neural fatigue mechanism

The most widely accepted theory of the mechanism behind the disorder is "neural fatigue". A motor unit is a nerve cell (or neuron) and the muscle fibers it activates. Poliovirus attacks specific neurons in the brainstem and the anterior horn cells of the spinal cord, generally resulting in the death of a substantial fraction of the neurons controlling skeletal muscles. In an effort to compensate for the loss of these neurons, surviving motor neurons sprout new nerve terminals to the orphaned muscle fibers. The result is some recovery of movement and the development of enlarged motor units.

The neural fatigue theory proposes that the enlargement of the motor neuron fibers places added metabolic stress on the nerve cell body to nourish the additional fibers. After years of use, this stress may be more than the neuron can handle, leading to the gradual deterioration of the sprouted fibers and, eventually, the neuron itself. This causes muscle weakness and paralysis. Restoration of nerve function may occur in some fibers a second time, but eventually nerve terminals malfunction and permanent weakness occurs. When these neurons no longer carry on sprouting, fatigue occurs due to the increasing metabolic demand of the nervous system. The normal aging process also may play a role. There is an ongoing denervation and reinnervation, but the reinnervation process has an upper limit where the reinnervation cannot compensate for the ongoing denervation, and loss of motor units takes place. However, what disturbs the denervation-reinnervation equilibrium and causes peripheral denervation is still unclear. With age, most people experience a decrease in the number of spinal motor neurons. Because polio survivors have already lost a considerable number of motor neurons, further age-related loss of neurons may contribute substantially to new muscle weakness. The overuse and underuse of muscles also may contribute to muscle weakness.

2-Auto immune reaction mechanism
Another theory is that people who have recovered from polio lose remaining healthy neurons at a faster rate than normal. However, little evidence exists to support this idea.[9] Finally, it has been proposed that the initial polio infection causes an autoimmune reaction, in which the body's immune system attacks normal cells as if they were foreign substances.

Physical problems of post-polio syndrome:

1-Slowly progressive muscle weakness
2-Muscle atrophy gradual decrease in the size of muscles
3- Pain from joint degeneration and increasing skeletal deformities
4-Fatigue (both generalized and muscu
5-Joint instability
6- Problems breathing or swallowing
7- Sleep-related breathing disorders, such as sleep apnea
8- Decreased tolerance for cold temperatures are other notable symptoms
9-Dysphagia (difficult in swallowing) Weakness in swallowing muscles can result in aspiration of food and liquids into the lungs and lead to pneumonia.

10-Dysarthria (difficulty in speaking)

11-Difficulty in ADL activities (feeding, dressing, toileting)

12-Respiratory muscle weakness-

13-Scoliosis increase of lateral curvature of the spine -

Treatment of post-polio syndrome:

The treatment for post-polio syndrome is enerally palliative and consists of and utilisation of mechanisms to make life easier such. In some cases, the use of lower limb orthotics can reduce energy usage.

1- Rest, analgesia (pain relief)

2- Energy conservation by

- Powered wheelchairs.

- Lifestyle changes

3- Reduce fatigue episodes

- reducing workload and daytime sleeping

4-Non fatigue muscle strength and endurance training are more important in managing the symptoms of PPS than the ability to perform long aerobic activity.

5- Hydrotherapy and developing other routines that encourage strength but do not affect fatigue levels

6-Electric stimulation for decreasing atrophy

7-Rthoses to prevent joint deterioration

8- Breathing exercises, chest percussion to remove secretions

9-Mild, decent and gentle stretching of tight muscles of scoliosis and lower limb muscle tightness

10- Weight loss is also recommended if patients areobese

11-Ocupational therapy training to enhance ADL activities

12-Speech therapy training to enhance swallowing and speech

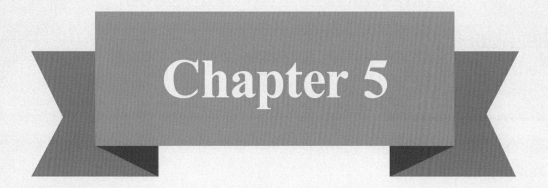

Chapter 5

Human genetics

- Medical genetics
- Genetic mutation (Muscular dystrophy)
- Autism
- Precautions in pediatric rehabilitation

Principles of medical genetics

Human genetics:
The science of variation and heredity in human beings.

The human chromosome
- Chromosomes are the elements inside nucleus which carry the genetic information
- Their number is constant (46 chromosome in human) composed of double helical DNA chain on a framework of protein

The number of chromosomes per cell varies in different species:

Chromosome Number for Selected Species: Table: (13)

Species	2n
Human being (Homo sapiens)	46
Garden pea (Pisum sativum)	14
Fruit fly (Drosophila melanogaster)	8
House mouse (Mus musculus)	40
Roundworm (Ascaris sp.)	2
Pigeon (Columba livia)	80
Boa constrictor (Constrictor constrictor)	36
Cricket (Gryllus domesticus)	22
Lily (Mum longiflorum)	24
Indian fern (Ophioglossum reticulatum)	1,260

- Segments of DNA molecules are called genes which are the units of heredity.
- Each gene has a precise position on a specific chromosome known as locus

Chromosomes & Genes

Are long stable DNA strands with many genes.

Occur in pairs in diploid organisms.

The two chromosomes in a pair are called "**homologs**"

Homologs usually contain the same genes, arranged in the same order

Homologs often have different alleles of specific genes that differ in part of their DNA sequence.

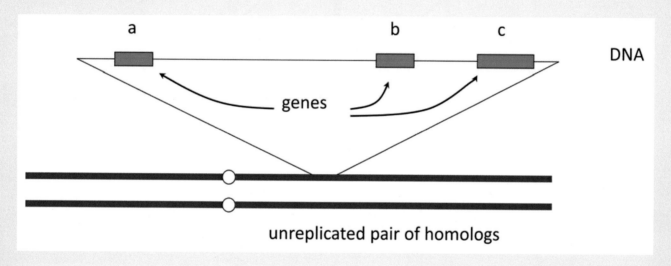

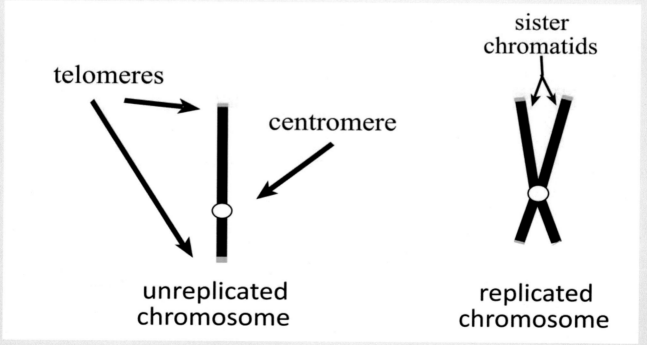

Fig (22): Chromosomes & Genes

Each chromatid consists of a very long strand of DNA. The DNA is Roughly colinear with the chromosome but is highly structured around Histones and other proteins which serve to condense its length and Control the activity of genes.

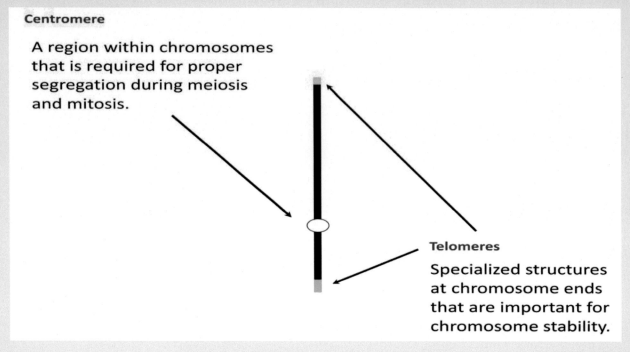

Fig (23): Structure of chromatide

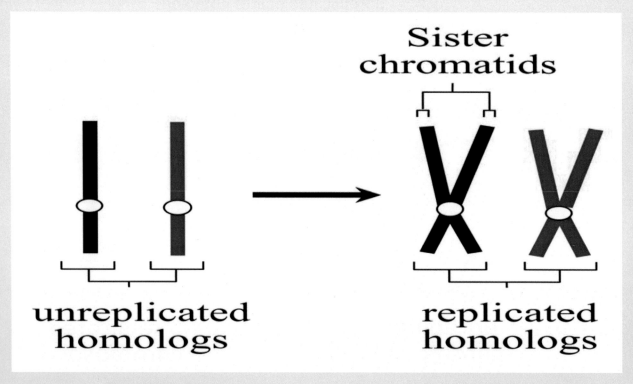

Fig (24): Replicated and unreplicated chromosomes

All human cells derived from single cell called zygote which has 46 chromosome formed by fertilization of ovum (23chr.) by sperm (23chr.) so all mother human cells contain 46chr.

Types of human cells:
- **Somatic cells**: all body cells except gonads. Divided by mitosis division giving 2 daughter cells has the same number of mother cell 46chr.
- **Germinal cells**: present only in gonads (ovary&testis) divided by meiosis producing 4cells

Comparision between mitosis and meiosis division: Table: (14)

Mitosis	Meiosis
One Division	Two Divisions
Homologues do not pair	Homologues Pair up
Centromeres divide	In meiosis I, centromeres do not divide
Each cell inherits both homologues	Homologues segregate from each other
Mitosis is conservative producing daughter cells that are like parental cell.	Meiosis is not conservative, rather it promotes variation through segregation of chromosomes and recombination

- In testis all 4 cells will form sperms each one contain 23 chr (half of the mother cell)
- In ovary only one ovum is formed at a time while the remaining will form polar bodies which will disintegrate

Type chromosomes:
Autosomes: 2x 22=44
Sex chr.: 2 i.e xx and xy

Mechanism of chromosomal aberration:

1-Non-disjunction: failure of separation of chromatids in mitosis division at the centromere this result in 2 daughter cells one with extra chr. And the other one less

2-Breakage:part of chromosome is broken with the result of:

- Deletion
- Translocation
- Iinversion
- Ring chromosome

3-Isochromosome formation: instead of longitudinal division of chr.

- Transverse division at centromere occur forming two identical parts one from two short arms the other from two long arms

Causes of chromosomal aberrations:

1-Old maternal age: over 35 years

2-Viral infection

3-Radiation

4-Drugs

5-Some chr. Aberration predispose to another aberration

Medical genetics deals with human genetic variation of medical significance. Major recognized areas of specialization are the study of chromosomes, and the structure and function of individual genes.

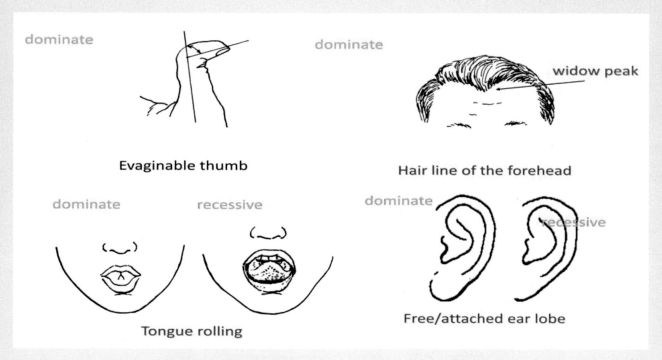

Fig (24): Dominant and recessive traits

Problems with doing human genetics:

Can't make controlled crosses!

Long generation time

Small number of offspring per cross

So, human genetics uses different methods

Chief method used in human genetics is pedigree analysis
I.e., the patterns of distribution of traits:

Pedigrees give information on:

Dominance or recessiveness of alleles

Risks (probabilities) of having affected offspring

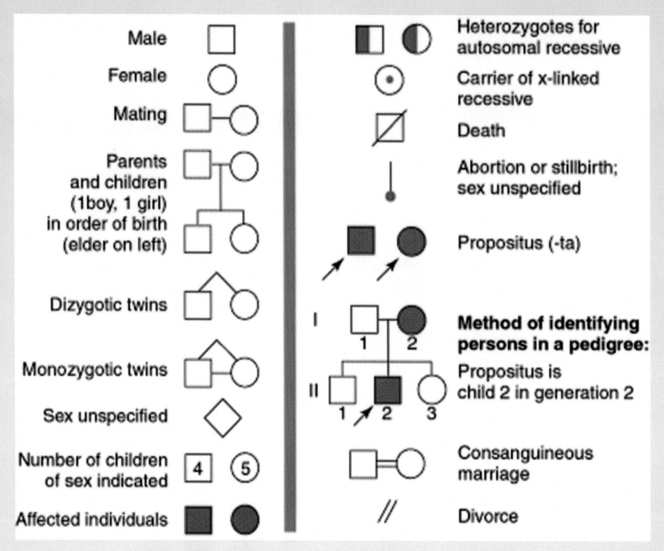

Fig (25): Standard symbols used in pedigrees

Genetic disease in Humans:

A. What is genetic disorder?

A genetic disorder is a disease that is caused by an abnormality in an individual's DNA. Abnormalities can range from a small mutation in a single gene to the addition or subtraction of an entire chromosome or set of chromosomes.

B. Characteristics of genetic disorders

1. Congenital
2. Mode of inheritance
3. Population distribution
4. Familial
5. Infectious

C. Classification of Genetic Disorders
1. Single-gene disorders
2. Chromosome disorders
3. Multi-factorial disorders
4. Somatic cell genetic disorders
5. Mitochondrial disorders

1-Single gene disorders
Single-gene disorders result when a mutation causes the protein product of a single gene to be altered or missing.

Single mutant gene has a large effect on the patient

Transmitted in a Mendelian fashion

Autosomal dominant, autosomal recessive, X-linked, Y-linked

Osteogenesis imperfecta - autosomal dominant

Sickle cell anaemia - autosomal recessive

Haemophilia - X-linked

2-Chromosomal disorders
In chromosome disorders, entire chromosomes, or large segments of them, are missing, duplicated, or otherwise altered.

Addition or deletion of entire chromosomes or parts of chromosomes

Typically more than 1 gene involved

1% of paediatric admissions and 2.5% of childhood deaths

Classic example is trisomy 21 - Down syndrome

3-Multi-factorial disorders
Multiple genes are missing as a result of this deletion, and each may contribute to the symptoms of the disorder. result from mutations in multiple genes, often coupled with environmental causes.

4-Somatic cell genetic diseases:
Result from the altered genetic materials in somatic cells.

5-Mitochondrial genetic diseases:
Due to the mutation of mitochondrial DNA.

-Role of Genes in Human Disease

Most diseases / phenotypes result from the interaction between genes and the environment

Some phenotypes are primarily genetically determined

Achondroplasia

Other phenotypes require genetic and environmental factors

Mental retardation in persons with PKU

Some phenotypes result primarily from the environment or chance

Lead poisoning

Short limbs, a normal-sized head and body, normal intelligence

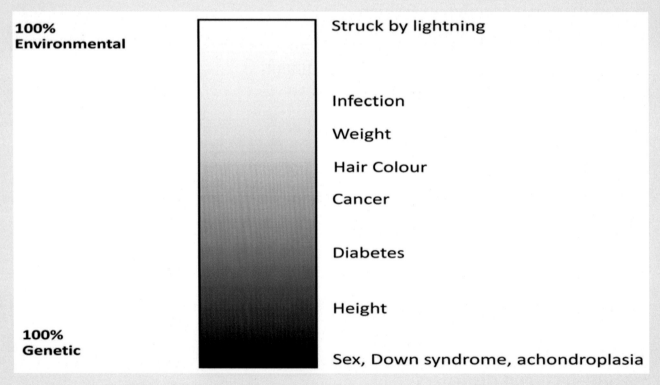

Fig (26): genetic and environmental contributions

Summary of mutations which can cause a disease

Single-base changes

Deletions/Insertions (indels)

Unstable repeat units

Two main effects

Loss of function

Gain of function

Three principal types of mutation:
- **Genetic Linkage disorder**
- **Mapping a disease Locus**
- **Linkage disorder**

Although Mendel's Law of Independent Assortment applies well to genes that are on different chromosomes. It does not apply well to two genes that are close to each other on the same chromosome.

Such genes are said to be "linked" and tend to segregate together in crosses.

Definitions:

Locus - a chromosomal location

Alleles - alternative forms of the same locus

Mutation - a change in the genetic material, usually rare and pathological

Polymorphism - a change in the genetic material, usually common and not pathological

Dominant trait - a trait that shows in a heterozygote

Recessive trait - a trait that is hidden in a heterozygote

<u>Muscular Dystrophies</u>

<u>Underlying mechanism of characteristics and physical problems in muscular dystrophy:</u>

The muscular dystrophy is distinguished from all other neuromuscular diseasesby

- Obligatory criteria:

(1) It is a Iry myopathy .

(2) There is a genetic basis for the disorder.

(3) The course is progressive.

(4) Degeneration and death of muscle fibers occur at some stage in the disease.

Duchenne Muscular Dystrophy

It is the most common hereditary neuromuscular disease.

Genetics: The gene is the DNA that encodes for a protein (dystrophin) necessary for the influx of ca++ via the sarcolemmal membranes of skeletal muscles, cardiac muscles, and also in the brain

Pathology of muscular dystrophy:

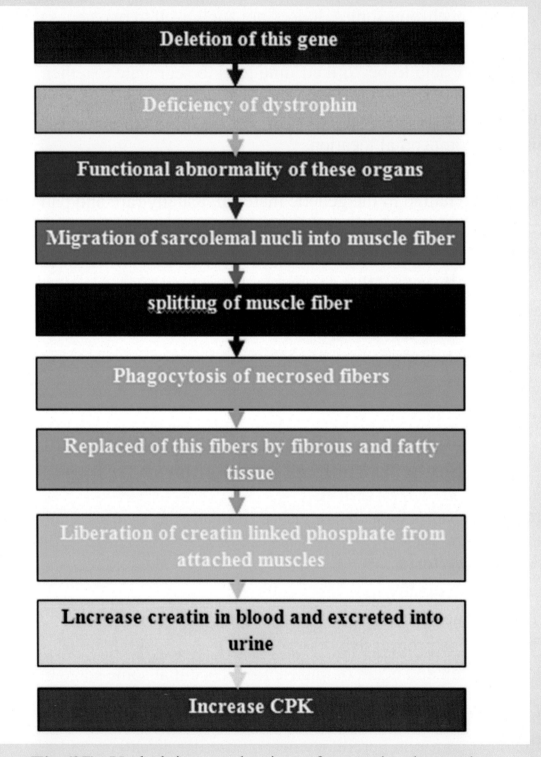

Fig (27): Underlying mechanism of muscular dystrophy

Clinical manifestation

1- During infancy:

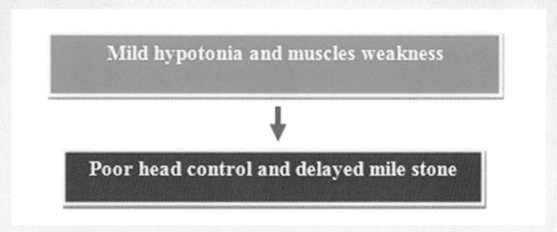

Fig (28): Cause of delaying mile stone in muscular dystrophy

2- During childhood:
A- Skeletal muscles disorders
1- Weakness: bilateral and symmetrical affection proximal more than distal:
Table: (15)

Muscle weaken	Result
-Pharyngealweakness	Episodes of aspiration
- Respiratory muscles	Frequent pulmonary infection
-Shoulder muscles	Cannot raise his hand
-Serratus anterior	Winging of the scapula
-Extensors of the trunk	Hyper lordosis of the spine
- Anterior abdominal muscles	Protuberant Abdomen
- Gluteus medius	Waddling gait
- Gluteus maximums	Gower sign

2- Hypotonia and hypo-reflexia the proximal reflexes less brisk than distal one
3- Pseudo-hypertrophy of calf and forearm muscles, atrophy of thigh muscles
4- Shortening of ankle muscles, knee muscles, hips and elbow muscles

B- Cardiomyopathy occur in early stage

C-Learning disability

D-No sensory manifestation

Prognosis: death occur perior to 20 years

Evaluation
1- History taken

2- Observation

3- Formal evaluation

4- Test of muscle tone

5- Test of tightness

6- Functional muscle test

7- Developmental stage test

Laboratory finding
1- Increase serum CPK

2- Increase lysosomal enzyme

3- ECG

4- EMG

5- NCV

6-Muscle biopsy

7- Genetic studies

Treatment
1- Facilitation of mile stone

2- Balance training

3- Active free ex

4- Gait training

5- Gentle stretch

6- Calcium intake

7- Myoplast transfer

8-Digoxin-antibiotic ss

Autism

Underlying mechanism of characteristics and behavior in autism:

Autism is a lifelong
g developmental disability that affects how a person communicates with, and relates to, other people and how they make sense of the world
around them.

Causes of Autism

- Genetic factor

There is no one cause of autism just as there is no one type of autism. Over the last five years, scientists have identified a number of rare gene changes, or mutations, associated with autism. A small number of these are sufficient to cause autism. Most cases of autism, however, appear to be caused by a combination of autism risk genes and environmental factors influencing early brain development.

- Environmental factors

In the presence of a genetic predisposition to autism, a number of non-genetic, or "environmental," stresses appear to further increase a child's risk. The clearest evidence of these autism risk factors involves events before and during birth. They include advanced parental age at time of conception (both mom and dad), maternal illness during pregnancy and certain difficulties during birth, particularly those involving periods of oxygen deprivation to the baby's brain. It is important to keep in mind that these factors, by themselves, do not cause autism. Rather, in combination with genetic risk factors, they appear to modestly increase risk.

A growing body of research suggests that a woman can reduce her risk of having a child with autism by taking prenatal vitamins containing folic acid and/or eating a diet rich in folic acid (at least 600 mcg a day) during the months before and after conception

Different names for autism

Some professionals may refer to autism by a different name, such as autism or autistic spectrum disorder (ASD), classic autism or Kanner autism, pervasive developmental disorder (PDD) or high-functioning autism (HFA).

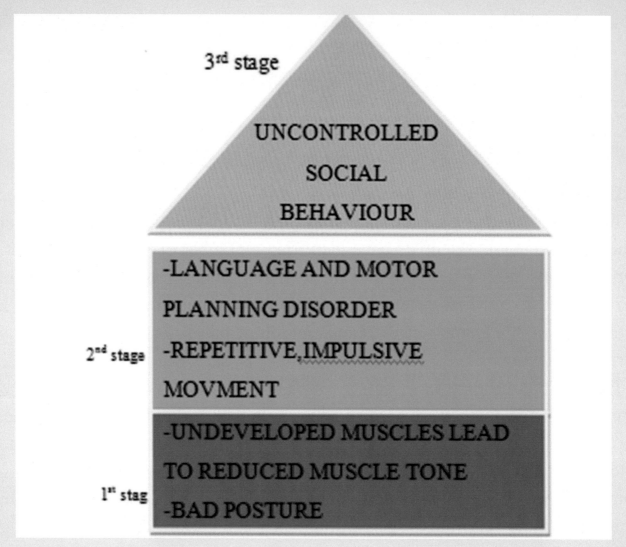

Fig.29): Stages of motor disorders in autism

Treatment of Autism

Common autism treatments include behavior therapy, speech-language therapy, play-based therapy, physical therapy, occupational therapy, and nutritional therapy. There is no cure for autism; however, with appropriate treatment and education, many children with autism spectrum disorders can learn and develop. Early intervention often can reduce challenges associated with autism, lessen disruptive behavior, and provide some degree of independence Treatment depends on the needs of the individual. In most cases, a combination of treatment methods is more effective. Autism spectrum disorders may require lifelong treatment. Speech therapy can help a child with autism improve language and social skills to communicate more effectively. physical therapy can help improve any deficiencies in coordination and motor skills. Occupational therapy may also help a child with autism to learn to process information from the senses (sight, sound, hearing, touch, and smell) in more manageable ways.

- Behavioral management therapy
- Cognitive behavior therapy
- Early intervention
- Educational and school-based therapies
- Joint attention therapy
- Medication treatment
- Nutritional therapy
- Occupational therapy
- Parent-mediated therapy
- Physical therapy
- Social skills training
- Speech-language therapy

Sensory Integration Therapy

Is a type of behavior modification that focuses on helping people with autism spectrum disorders cope with sensory stimulation. Treatment may include having the individual handle materials with different textures or listen to different sounds .Sensory integration therapy helps the person deal with sensory information, like sights, sounds, and smells. Sensory integration therapy could help a child who is bothered by certain sounds or does not like to be touched

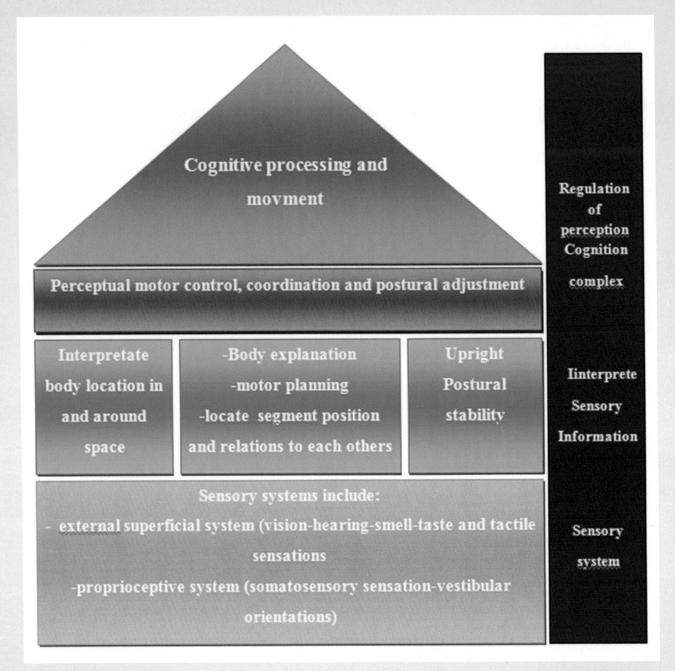

Fig. 30): Sensory systems as a foundation of movment in autism

Speech and language therapy (SLT) is a type of skills training designed to improve your child's language skills. This can improve their ability to interact with others socially. The therapist uses a number of techniques, such as visual aids, stories and toys, to improve communication skills

Makaton is a communication programmed where signs and symbols are used to help people with ASD communicate with others. The signs used in Makaton are based on British Sign Language (BSL), and each sign has a corresponding symbol. These symbols are simple drawings that can often be used independently of the signs. The signs or symbols can be used with speech to help provide extra clues about what someone is saying. Over time, as their speech and language skills develop, many people with ASD will gradually stop using the signs or symbols and start to rely more on their speech to communicate. Makaton can be helpful for improving basic communication in some people with ASD, as well as helping improve social interaction an Makaton can be helpful for improving basic communication in some people with ASD, as well as helping improve social interaction and the ability to build relationships.

.Dietary Approaches

Some dietary treatments have been developed by reliable therapists. But many of these treatments do not have the scientific support needed for widespread recommendation. An unproven treatment might help one child, but may not help another. Many biomedical interventions call for changes in diet. Such changes include removing certain types of foods from a child's diet and using vitamin or mineral supplements. Dietary treatments are based on the idea that food allergies or lack of vitamins and minerals cause symptoms of ASD. Some parents feel that dietary changes make a difference in how their child acts or feels. Researchers have found elevated levels of proteins found in wheat, oats and rye (gluten) and casein (protein in dairy products) by-products in people with autism, suggesting that the incomplete breakdown or excessive absorption of these substances may affect brain function. Eliminating foods that contain gluten and casein from the diet may cause **side effects** and should not be done without the advice of a qualified health care provider.

Studies have shown that vitamin B, magnesium (improves the effects of vitamin B), and cod liver oil supplements (which contain vitamins A and D) may improve behavior, eye contact, attention span, and learning in autistic people. Vitamin C has been shown to improve depression and lessen the severity of symptoms in people with autism

Behavioral training and management:

Uses positive reinforcement, self-help, and social skills training to improve behavior and communication. Many types of treatments have been developed, including Applied Behavioral Analysis (ABA), sensory integration and Treatment and Education of Autistic and Related Communication Handicapped Children (TEACCH) whichis a type of educational intervention that emphasizes structured learning by using visual prompts. Research has found children with ASD often respond better to information that's presented visually. TEACCH is often delivered at special day centres, but you can also have training so you can continue the intervention activities at home. There are several methods of behavior modification that are used to treat inappropriate, repetitive, and aggressive behavior and to provide autistic people with skills necessary to function in their environment. Most types of behavior modification are based on the theory that rewarded behavior is more likely to be repeated than behavior that is ignored. This theory is called applied behavior analysis (ABA).

Applied behavior analysis (ABA) involves breaking down skills, such as communication and cognitive skills, into small tasks and teaching those tasks in a highly structured way. It also rewards and reinforces positive behavior while discouraging inappropriate behaviour.ABA sessions are usually carried out at home, although some programmes can be integrated into schools or nurseries. An ABA programme usually begins with simple tasks that become more complex over time, which can help your child's development by gradually improving their skills. Behavior modification often involves highly structured, skill-oriented activities that are based on the individual's needs and interests. It usually requires intense, one-on-one training with a therapist and extensive caregiver involvement. Social interaction is often affected by limited emotional development that is common in autistic people.

Play therapy is a type of behavior modification that is used to improve emotional development, which in turn, improves social skills and learning. Play therapy involves adult-child interaction that is controlled by the child.

Social stories can also be used to improve undeveloped social skills. Stories are designed to help people with autism spectrum disorders understand the feelings, ideas, and points of view of others, or to suggest an alternate response to a particular situation. They also may be used to help people with autism understand and cope with their own feelings. Behavioral therapists can teach caregivers how to develop social stories.

Parent education and training, Communication advice for parents and Parent support programmes the parents of a child with ASD play a crucial role in supporting their child and helping improve their skills.
Communication is particularly challenging for children with ASD. Helping your child communicate can lead to reduced anxiety and improved behaviour.

The following tips may be useful when
- Communicating and interacting with your child:
- Use your child's name so they know you're addressing them
- Keep background noise to a minimum
- Keep language simple
- Speak slowly and clearly with pauses between words
- Accompany what you say with simple gestures
- Allow extra time for your child to process what you've said
For more in-depth advice, programmes specifically designed to help parents of children recently diagnosed with ASD are available

Psychological therapy If your child's behavior is causing problems, they'll be assessed for possible triggers, such as a physical health condition, mental health problem, or environmental factors. In cases where a child with ASD also has a mental health problem, such as anxiety, a psychological treatment may be offered.
Psychological treatments, such as cognitive behavioral therapy (CBT), involve talking to a therapist about thoughts and feelings, and discussing how these affect behavior and wellbeing. If a treatment like CBT is offered, the therapist should be aware of any changes or adaptations that need to be made to the therapy because of the ASD. This might include using more written or visual information – for example, worksheets and images – and using plain English

Autism Prognosis People with autism have normal life expectancies. With early intervention and appropriate treatment, many autistic people can function productively and attain some degree of independence. Some people with autism spectrum disorders require lifelong assistance.

Any intervention should focus on important aspects of your child's development these are:
- **Communication skills** – such as the ability to start conversations
- **Social interaction skills** – such as the ability to understand other people's feelings and respond to them
- **Cognitive (thinking) skills** – such as encouraging imaginative play
- **Academic skills** – the "traditional" skills a child needs to progress with their education, such as reading, writing and maths.

Precautions in pediatric rehabilitation

Underlying mechanism of methods, techniques and physical problems in different cases in pediatric rehabilitation

1-In applications of faradic stimulation:
- Stimulation of anti-spastic muscles as stimulations of ant-tibial group to inhibit spasticity of calf muscles in this situation we should support ankle in dorsiflexion position due to the spastic muscles are hypersensitive to electric stimulation more than antispastic so without support of ankle we stimulate calf spastic muscles not the anti spastic one(no gain of relaxation of spastic muscles)

2-In applications of U.S:
- It is forbidden to apply U.S end of the bone(on the joint) because mechanical waves will destruct the metaphysis which is responsible for bone growth

- In torticollus U.S applied away from trachea because mechanical waves produce injuries to trachea cartilage .we should apply pulsed U.S on and around muscle mass only
- Continuous U.S used in tightness on bulky muscles for increase of elasticity and improve circulation and on strained, not odemeatus muscles
- Pulsed U.S (no associated heat) used in odemeatus strained muscles as in torticollus

3-Electric stimulation contra-indications in pediatric
- On spastic muscles
- Epilepsy
- Vomiting
- Fever
- Headache (sever crying)

4-Main indication of electric stimulationk
- Atrophy is the problem we looking for when we want to use faradic stimulation in pediatric
- In LMNL atrophy must occur so in more than 90% of LMNL need faradic stimulation
- In UMNL atrophy not occurred except in neglectionbut we use it for inhibition of spastic by stimulation faradic on anti-spastic muscles (produce reciprocal inhibition)

5-In applications of short wave
- We use small cups,3 towels rounding area of application, remove any type of metals and avoid wire crossing
- In pediatric we use prolonged time (20 minutes) and lowest power(1 or 2 grade)
- In diabetes we use prolonged time (20 minutes) and lowest power(1 or 2 grade) due to peripheral neuritis and sensory affection

6-laser applications in pediatric
- scanned laser can be used for treating bedsores
- probe laser can be used for proliferation of ATP

help in nerve regeneration as in Bells palsy in front and bellow earand in Erbs palsy on erbs point in lower third of sternoclidomastoid muscle just behind clavicle

7-On application of infra –red
- Eyes must be protected from infra red rays when we apply I.R on sound side for relaxation

8-Passive stretch precautions
- Mild gentle and decent stretch must be used
- Limiting factors are crying of the child, facial expression resistance and limitation of movement
- Over correction of tight muscle lead to muscle strain

9-Approximation
- Applied in all range of the joint to stimulate all proprioceptors of the joint
- Approximation of the head must be slow in spastic,hypotonic and fluctuating muscles to avoid sprain in neck ligament
- Slow, rhythmic approximation used in spasticity inhibition
- Rapid, un rhythmic approximation used in facilitation of Hypotonia
- Jerky approximation used in fluctuating hypertonia
- Hand cupping over anterior fontanelles should be performed to avoid its injury

10 –precautions in hydrocephalus
- Approximation of head in hydrocephalus by cupping of head at ear and slow approximation
- Hydrocephalus and congenital heart disease child don't put them in upside down on ball
- Parachut reaction training don't perform in hydrocephalus

11-Myopathy
- Don't use resistance ex. to avoid fatigue and exhusion
- Active free ex must be used

12-Erb's palsy

- Stretching ex of sub scapularis muscles must be applied in complete adducted shoulder to avoid subluxation

13-In all pediatric cases

- Hip stability tests must be performed at first to exclude CDH to avoid fractures due to osteoporosis from bed ridden complication specially old cerebral palsy children

14-Spina bifida

- Sensation lost should be in your mind when you apply brief icing or heat

15- Cerebral palsy

- Involuntary movement associated with laxity of ligament and hyper-mobility of the joints mobilization is forbidden and weight bearing ex should be with splint to avoid deformity
- Over stretch produce fracture due to osteoporosis

16- Post-operative cases

- Don't use short wave or US over plate and screw fixation
- Don't use dynamic ex in cruciate ligament reconstruction operationbut use isometric ex

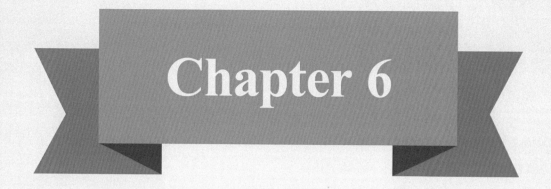

Chapter 6

(Developmental psychology)

- Definitions of terms
- language, speech and writing skills acquisition:
- Personality development
- Cognitive development

Human growth and development:
Changes that all human being face across their life span

Changes comes from: Increase age, experience, genetic potentials and interactions of all three factors

Domains of human development
1-Cognetive (learning of new skills)
2-Motor(development of human movement)
3-Affective(emotional and social development)
4-Physical(body changes)

Elements of developmental changes
Qualitative, sequential, cumulative, directional, multifactorial, individual

Definitions
Development: Interactional process that lead to behavioral changes over life span
Growth:
Quantitative structural changes of development Maturations: qualitative functional changes of development

Development include both growth and maturation

Specific cortical area:
Frontal lobe: Voluntary motor activity, storage of motor pattern, language, motor speech

Parietal lobe: Processing of sensory input
Occipital: Visual receptive area
Temporal: Auditory and speech receptive area

<u>Under lying mechanism of language, speech and writing skills acquisition:</u>

Sound enter to outer canal to ear canal to ear drum which transfer sound to mechanical waves to air filled space(middle ear) vibration transmitted to inner ear(fluid filled cochlea)Vibration push into cochlea lead to disturbance fluid lead to wave set up travel via vestibulochlear nerve tocochlear nuclous, superior olivary complex of brain stem to thalamus(feeling of sound)to temporal lobe(area22)understanding of spoken words and to occipit lobe Understanding of written wordarea18,19 all those information go to wrinkles area in temporal lobe(general interpretation area) and from area5,7 somatic sensory arear of paraital lobe sending them to brocas area which make motor command to cortico-bulbar tractto cranial nerve nuclii to speech musclesAlso sending them to exners area(writing motor center) to cortico-spinal tract to A.H.C. to hand muscle .

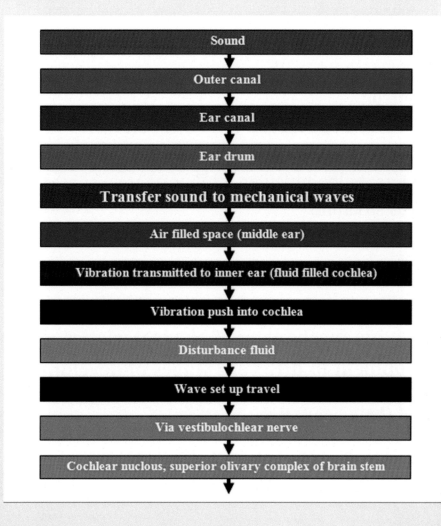

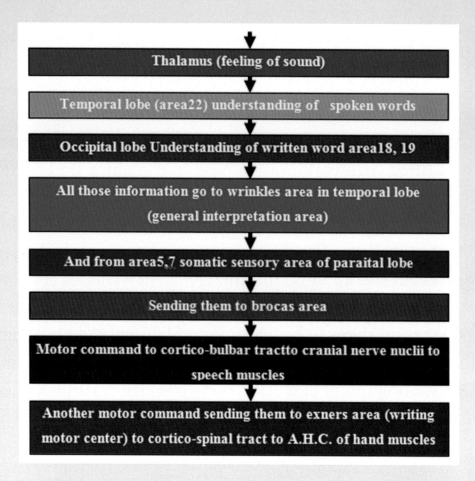

Fig.31): Underlying mechanism of speech, language and writing skills acquisition

Supra-spinal control:

1-Facilitatory centers: bulbo-reticular facilitatory area, area 4,vestibular nuclus, neocerebellum

2-Inhibitory centers: bulbo reticular inhibitory area, supressor areas, paleo cerebellum, corpus striatum

Personality development

Underlying mechanism of characteristics and its development in different stages of development

1-Critical period (babyhood) 0-2

Foundations of personality structure built in due to:

1-Affected by emotional deprivation as neglect in home

2-Limited environment the mother is the most constant companion

3-Active stage of independence when subjected to overprotection cause its failure

4-Sex difference produce environmental pressure which increase with time

5-Genetic factor which affect on personality traits, pattern

Family causes lead to personality changes

1-Degree of dependence:

increase of it lead to increase appealing

2-Parental anxiety: increase of anxiety on baby become negativistic, crying excessively

3-Child training methods: permissive or authoritarian corporal punishment associated with authority damage parent child relationship

4-Maternal employment: mother work baby will have strong emotional attachment with servant of home resentment parent child relation ship

5-Maternal overwork: mother become tense, nervous, irritable in unfavorable situation

6-Arrival of new sibling: child sense of neglection

7-Preference of certain family member

Personality changes in this stage is quantitative (strength or weak of trait) and qualitative (change of undesirable trait to desirable one)

II-Early childhood

Family relationship- core of self concept

core of personality pattern which take form in this period

- Enviroment here (parents, siblings, relatives, peers, neighborhood, child care center)

- Attitude of their peers, ways of their peers treat them affect on self concept

Factors shaping self concept:

1- Parents attitude toward his abilities, behaviour

2-Child training method: strict, authoritarian behavior associated with corporal punishment lead to martyr complex

3-Aspiration of parents:

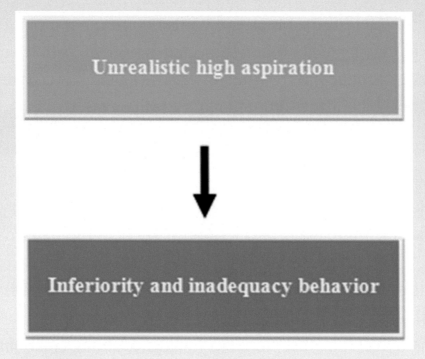

Fig.32): Effect of parent aspiration on the child personality

4-Ordinal position of children: each child in family play a specific role
5-Sex role identification: boys with masculine physiques more successful in interacting with other boys
6-Enviromental insecurity: death, divorce, separation sense difference from peers

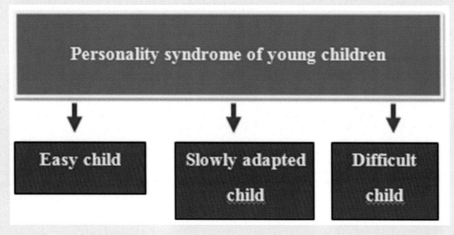

Fig.33): Types of child personality

Easy child: well adjusted physically and psychologically
Slow adapted child: low activity level, don't adapt quickly
Difficult child: intense in reaction

Types of personality:
- Leader-follower
- Despotic-meek
- Sociable-solitary
- Center of attention-shun
- Egocentric-conformer

III-Late childhood

Factors affecting self concept:

1-Physical condition: poor health off from playing with peers lead to sense of inferiority

2-Body build: overweight or very small felling of inferiority

3-Names and nicknames: names which suggest minority and fun lead to inferiority

4-Socio economic status: better homes, betterclothes, betterplay equipment

5-School enviroment: unfair, aggressive teacher lead to undiscipline behaviour

6--Social acceptance: very popular and isolates are the result

7-Success and failure: success lead to self confidence, acceptance

8-Sex: society evaluation of girls as inferior and so value themselves less

9-Intellegence: below average sense inferiority very high IQ sense poor self concept due to adult expect more and more from them

IV-Adolescent

- Factor affecting on self concept

1-Age of maturation: early matures good adjustments behavior late matures maladjusted behavior

2-Appearance: being different feel inferiority (either in clothes or physical dysfunction)

3-Sex-appropriateness:sex appropriate appearance lead to favorable self concept

4-Names and nicknames: if peer group judge name unfavorable effect occur

5-Family relationship: close relationship with member lead todevelop similar personality pattern

6-Peers reflections of what they believes, their concepts also child under the peers pressures to develop personality traits approved to the group

7-Creativity: child who encouraged to be creative in play and academic work develop individuality which has positive effect on self concept

8-Level of aspiration: unrealistic high levels of aspiration lead to failure and opposite.

Cognitive Development

Underlying mechanism of cognition development:

Intelligence was not random, but was a set of organized cognitive structures that the infant actively constructed (interaction between genetic factor+ environmental factor)

This construction occurs through the adaptation to the environment

Adaptation: Two Mechanisms

Assimilation: Interpreting or construing environmental events in terms of one's existing cognitive structures and ways of thinking

Accommodation: Changing one's existing cognitive structures and ways of thinking to apprehend environmental events

Stages of cognitive Development

- Development of qualitatively different cognitive structures occurred through the processes of assimilation and accommodation.
- When a qualitative change occurs, the infant/child enters a new stage of development

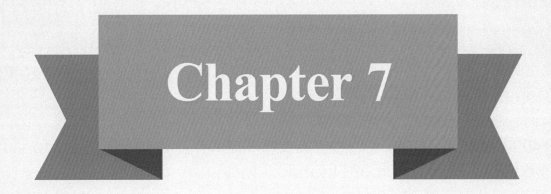

Chapter 7

<u>References (for further reading)</u>

1-Abbeduto, Leonard; Ozonoff, Susan; Thurman, Angela John; McDuffie, Angela; Schweitzer, Julie. Hales, Robert; Yudofsky, Stuart; Robert, Laura Weiss, eds. 2015Chapter 8. Neurodevelopmental Disorders, The American Psychiatric Publishing Textbook of Psychiatry (6 ed.). Arlington, VA: American Psychiatric Publishing. ISBN 978-1-58562-444-7. Retrieved 11 March.

2-Abernethy B, Sparrow WA. 1992Approaches to the Study of Motor Control and Learning. Amsterdam, the Netherlands: Elsevier Science; :3–45.

3-Amir, Ruthie; Van den Veyver, Ignatia; Wan, Mimi; Tran, Charles; Francke, Uta; Zoghbi, Huda (1999). "Rett syndrome. Nature Genetics **23** (2): 185–8. doi:10.1038/13810. PMID 10508514.

4-Barnes MJ, Johnson GS (2001) Upper Motor Neurone Syndrome and Spasticity. Arch Phys Med Rehabil 23: 453-460.

5-Bly L. 1991 A historical and current view of the basis of NDT. Pediatric Physical Therapy. ;3:131–135.

6-Bobath, B., 1967. The Very Early Treatment of Cerebral Palsy. Developmental Medicine and Child Neurology. 9, 373-390.

7-Bobath, B., Bobath, K., 1964. The Facilitation of Normal Postural Reactions and Movements in the Treatment of Cerebral Palsy. Physiotherapy, London.

8-Bobath, B., Bobath, K., 1984. The Neuro-Developmental Treatment. In: Scrutton, D., and al. Oxford, pp. 6-18

9-Boehme, R., 1988. Improving Upper Body Control. TherapySkill Builders, U.S.A., pp. 1-18.

10-Boschen KA, Wright FV. 1995 Assessment of the reliability and validity of the Pediatric Evaluation of Disability Inventory (PEDI). Veterans Health Administration Rehabilitation Research and Development Service. ; 32:60–61.

11-Bower E. 1993Physiotherapy for cerebral palsy: a historical review. In: Ward CD, eds. Rehabilitation of Motor Disorders. Baillièere's Clinical Neurology. Vol 2. London, England: Baillièere Tindall; :29–54.

12-Bower E. 1997The multiply handicapped child. In: Cambridge, England: Cambridge University Press; :315–356.

13-Bryce, J., 1972. Facilitation of Movement-the Bobath Approach. Physiotherapy. 58, 403-408.

14-Cookson JC. 1979 Orthopedic manual therapy an overview, pan 2: the spine. Phys Ther.; 59:259267.

15-Cools AM, Witvrouw EE, Danneels LA, *et al.* 2002 Does taping influence electromyographic muscle activity in the scapular rotators in healthy shoulders? Man Ther.;7:154–162.

16-Fetters L. 1991Measurement and treatment in cerebral palsy: an argument for a new approach. Phys Ther. ;71:244–247.

17-Fife S, Roxborough LA, Story M, Field D, Harris SR, Armstrong RW et al. (1993) Reliability of a measure to assess outcomes of adaptive seating in children with neuromotor disabilities. Can J Rehabil 7: 11-13.

18-Fife SE, Roxborough LA, Armstrong RW, Harris SR, Gregson JL, et al.(1991) Development of a clinical measure of postural control for assessment of adaptive seating in children with neuromotor disabilities. Phys Ther 71: 981-993.

19-Finnie, N.R., 1968. Handling the Young Child with Cerebral Palsy at Home. Butterworth-Heinemann, Oxford.

20-Finnie, N.R., 1997. Handling the Young Child with Cerebral Palsy at Home. Butterworth-Heinemann, Oxford. 3rd Ed.

21-Freeman, Michael D.; Rosa, Scott; Harshfield, David; Smith, Francis; Bennett, Robert; Centeno, Christopher J.; Kornel, Ezriel; Nystrom, Ake; Heffez, Dan; Kohles, Sean S. (2010). "A case-control study of cerebellar tonsillar ectopia (Chiari) and head/neck trauma (whiplash)". Brain Injury **24**(7-8): 988–94. doi: 10.3109/02699052.2010.490512. PMID 20545453.

22-Gramsbergen, A., Hadders-Algra, M., 1998. Development of Postural Control. Neuroscience & Biobehavioral Reviews. 22, 463-595.

23-Grieve GP. 1989 Contra-indications to spinal manipulation and allied treatments. Physiotherapy.;75:44953.

24-Guo CB, Zhang W, Ma DQ, Zhang KH, Huang JQ (1996) Hand grip strength: an indicator of nutritional state and the mix of postoperative complications in patients with oral and maxillofacial cancers. Br J Oral Maxillofac Surg 34: 325-327.

25-Hadders-Algra, M., 1996. The assessment of General Movements is a valuable technique for the detection of brain dysfunction in young infants. A review. Acta Paediatrica. Suppl 416, 39-43.

26-Haley SM, Coster WJ, Ludlow LH, et al. 1992Pediatric Evaluation of Disability Inventory (PEDI). Boston, Mass: New England Medical Center Hospitals .

27-Heriza C. 1991 Motor development: traditional and contemporary theories. In: Lister MJ, eds. Contemporary Management of Motor Control Problems: Proceedings of the II STEP Conference. Alexandria, Va: Foundation for Physical Therapy; :99–126.

28-Hirschfeld, H., 1992. Postural Control: Acquisition and Integration during Development. Movement Disorders in Children. Medicine and Sport Science 36, Karger, Basel, pp. 199-208.

29-Hochleitner, M., 1986. Das Bobath-Konzept. Der Kinderartzt.17, 539.

30-Horak FB. 1992 Motor control models underlying neurologic rehabilitation of posture in children. Movement Disorders in Children. Basel, Switzerland: Karger; :21–30.

31-Hur JJ. 1995Review of research on therapeutic interventions for children with cerebral palsy. Acta Neurol Scand. ;91:423–432.

32-Ingram TTS. 1984 A historical review of the definition and classification of the cerebral palsies.. London, England: Heinemann; :1–11.

33-Ivanhoe CB, Reistetter TA (2004) Spasticity: the misunderstood part of the upper motor neuron syndrome. Am J Phys Med Rehabil 83: S3-S9.

34-Jian, Le; Nagarajan, Lakshmi; De Klerk, Nicholas; Ravine, David; Bower, Carol; Anderson, Alison; Williamson, Sarah; Christodoulou, John; Leonard, Helen (2006). "Predictors of seizure onset in Rett syndrome". The Journal of Pediatrics **149** (4): 542–7. doi:10.1016/j.jpeds.2006.06.015. PMID 17011329.

35-Ketelaar M, van Petegem-van Beek E, Visser JJW. 1995Gross Motor Function Measure Manual: Nederlandse Vertaling. Utrecht, the Netherlands: Utrecht University .

36-Ketelaar M. 1999Children With Cerebral Palsy: A Functional Approach to Physical Therapy. Delft, the Netherlands: Eburon .

37-Kibler WB. 1998The role of the scapula in athletic shoulder function. Am JSports Med.;26:325–337.

38-Kuhn JE. 2003 Scapulothoracic crepitus and bursitis in athletes. In: orthopaedicsports medicine.2nd ed. Philadelphia: WB Saunders;: 1006–1014.

39-Kumar RT, Pandyan AD, Sharma AK (2006) Biomechanical measurement of post-stroke spasticity. Age Ageing 35: 371-375.

40-Kwon JM. Miscellaneous Disorders. In: Kliegman RM, Behrman RE, Jenson HB, Stanton BF, eds. 2011Nelson Textbook of Pediatrics. 19th ed. Philadelphia, PA: Saunders Elsevier;:chap 592.5.

41-Lashkari, A.; Smith, A. K.; Graham, J. M. (1999). "Williams-Beuren Syndrome: An Update and Review for the Primary Physician". Clinical Pediatrics **38** (4): 189–208. doi:10.1177/000992289903800401. PMID 10326175.

42-Lenhoff, Howard M.; Teele, Rita L.; Clarkson, Patricia M.; Berdon, Walter E. (2010). "John C. P. Williams of Williams-Beuren syndrome". Pediatric Radiology **41** (2): 267–9. doi:10.1007/s00247-010-1909-y. PMID 21107555.

43-Loukas M, Shayota BJ, Oelhafen K, Miller JH, Chern JJ, Tubbs RS, Oakes WJ (2011). "Associated disorders of Chiari Type I malformations: a review". Neurosurg Focus **31** (3): E3. doi:10.3171/2011.6.FOCUS11112. PMID 21882908.

44-Maitland GD. 1977Peripheral Manipulation. Boston, Mass: ButterworthPublishers.

45-Manske RC, Reiman MP, Stovak ML. 2004 Nonoperative and operativemanagement of snapping scapula. Am J Sports Med.;32: 1554–1565.

46-Martens, Marilee A.; Wilson, Sarah J.; Reutens, David C. (2008). "Research Review: Williams syndrome: A critical review of the cognitive, behavioral, and neuroanatomical phenotype". Journal of Child Psychology and Psychiatry **49** (6): 576–608. doi:10.1111/j.1469-7610.2008.01887.x. PMID 18489677.

47-McDonald RL, Surtees R (2007) Longitudinal study evaluating a seating system using a sacral pad and kneeblock for children with cerebral palsy. Disabil Rehabil 29: 1041-1047.

48-McDonnell MN, Hillier SL, Ridding MC, Miles TS (2006) Impairments in precision grip correlate with functional measures in adult hemiplegia. Clin Neurophysiol 117: 1474-1480.

49-Meijer OG, Roth K. 1988Complex Movement Behaviour: The Motor-Action Controversy. Amsterdam, the Netherlands: Elsevier Science; .

50-Mortenson WB, Miller WC, Auger C (2008) Issues for the selection of wheelchair-specific activity and participation outcome measures: a review. Arch Phys Med Rehabil 89: 1177-1186.

51-Nichols DS, Case-Smith J. 1996 Reliability and validity of the Pediatric Evaluation of Disability Inventory. Pediatric Physical Therapy.;8:15–24.

52-Piper MC, Darrah J. 1994Motor Assessment of the Developing Infant. Philadelphia, Pa: WB Saunders Co; .

53-Pohl M, Mehrholz J, Rockstroh G, Rückriem S, Koch R (2007) Contractures and involuntary muscle overactivity in severe brain injury. Brain Inj 21: 421- 432.

54-rancke, U. (1999). "Williams-Beuren syndrome: genes and mechanisms". Human Molecular Genetics **8** (10): 1947–54. doi:10.1093/hmg/8.10.1947. PMID 10469848.

55-Riveira, Carmiña; Pascual, Julio (2007). "Is Chiari type I malformation a reason for chronic daily headache?". Current Pain and Headache Reports **11** (1): 53–5. doi:10.1007/s11916-007-0022-x. PMID 17214922.

56-Rosenbaum, RB; DP Ciaverella (2004). Neurology in Clinical Practice. Butterworth Heinemann. pp. 2192–2193. ISBN 0-7506-7469-5.

57-Royeen CB, DeGangi GA. 1992 Use of neurodevelopmental treatment as an intervention: annotated listing of studies 1980-1990. Percept Motor Skills. ;75:175–194.

58-Russell D, Rosenbaum PL, Gowland C, et al. 1993Manual for the Gross Motor Function Measure. Hamilton, Ontario, Canada: McMaster University; .

59-Russell DJ, Rosenbaum PL, Cadman DT, et al. 1989 The Gross Motor Function Measure: a means to evaluate the effects of physical therapy. Dev Med Child Neurol. ;31:341–352.

60-Ryan, Monique M. (December 2013). "Pediatric Guillain-Barré syndrome". Current Opinion in Pediatrics **25** (6): 689–693. doi:10.1097/MOP.0b013e328365ad3f. PMID 24240288.

61-Safran MR. 2004 Nerve injury about the shoulder in athletes. Part 2. Longthoracic nerve, spinal accessory nerve, burners/stingers, thoracic outlet syndrome. Am J Sports Med.;32:1063–1076

62-Sartorius, G. A.; Nieschlag, E. (20 August 2009). "Paternal age and reproduction". Human Reproduction Update **16** (1): 65–79. doi:10.1093/humupd/dmp027. PMID 19696093.

63-Scrutton D. 1984Management of Motor Disorders of Children With Cerebral Palsy. Oxford, England: Blackwell Scientific; . Clinics in Developmental Medicine publication no. 90.

64-Shaw G.M., Carmichael S.L., Kaidarova Z., Harris J.A. (2003) Differential risks to males and females for congenital malformations among 2.5 million California births, 1989-1997. Birth Defects Res. A Clin. Mol. Teratol. **67(12)** p. 953-958.

65-Shepherd RB. 1995Physiotherapy in Paediatrics. Oxford, England: Butterworth-Heinemann; .

66-Shumway-Cook A, Anson D, Haller S (1988) Postural sway biofeedback: its effect on reestablishing stance stability in hemiplegic patients. Arch Phys Med Rehabil 69: 395-400.

67-Shumway-Cook A, Woollacott MH. 1995Motor Control: Theory and Practical Applications. Baltimore, Md: Williams & Wilkins; .

68-Stevenson TJ, Garland SJ (1996) Standing balance during internally produced perturbations in subjects with hemiplegia: validation of the balance scale. Arch Phys Med Rehabil 77: 656-662.

69-Tirosh E, Rabino S. 1989 Physiotherapy for children with cerebral palsy: evidence for its efficacy. Am J Dis Child. ;143:552–555.

70-Tsai, Luke Y. (1992). "Is Rett syndrome a subtype of pervasive developmental disorders?". Journal of Autism and Developmental Disorders **22** (4): 551–61. doi:10.1007/BF01046327. PMID 1483976.

71-van den Berg, Bianca; Walgaard, Christa; Drenthen, Judith; Fokke, Christiaan; Jacobs, Bart C.; van Doorknob, Pieter A. (15 July 2014). "Guillain–Barré syndrome: pathogenesis, diagnosis, treatment and prognosis". Nature Reviews Neurology **10** (8): 469–482. doi:10.1038/nrneurol.2014.121. PMID 25023340.

72-van Doorn, Pieter A; Ruts, Liselotte; Jacobs, Bart C (October 2008). "Clinical features, pathogenesis, and treatment of Guillain-Barré syndrome". The Lancet Neurology **7** (10): 939–950. doi:10.1016/S1474-4422(08)70215-1. PMID 18848313.

73-Wells PE. Manipulative procedures. In: Wells PE, Frampton V, Bowsher D, eds. 1988 Pain Management in Physical Therapy. East Norwalk,Conn: Appleton and Lange;:181--217.

74-Yuki, Nobuhiro; Hartung, Hans-Peter (14 June 2012). "Guillain–Barré Syndrome". New England Journal of Medicine **366** (24): 2294–2304. doi:10.1056/NEJMra1114525. PMID 22694000.

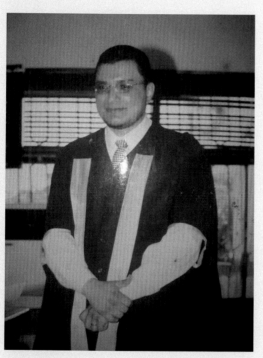

Dr.Ahmed Mohamed Azzam is an Egyptian assistant professor in pediatric rehabilitation from Mansoura city in the heart of the Niles Delta. Currently, he becomes ass. Professor in Department of phys iotherapy for developmental disturbance and pediatric surgery, Faculty of physical therapy, Cairo university, Egypt. Dr. Azzam has been awarded his PH.D degree in pediatric rehabilitation in Faculty of physical therapy; Cairo University, Egypt .He is holding a master degree in pediatric rehabilitation from Faculty of physical therapy, Cairo University, Egypt.

-After 10 years of hard work, he finally issued his series of rehabilitation (essential mechanisms of neurological pediatric rehabilitation, essential mechanisms of orthopedic pediatric rehabilitation and Azzam scale in practical guide to occupational therapy). Dr. Azzam aimed at making pediatric rehabilitation interesting and of direct application to physiotherapy and occupational therapy .In our books text is linked with graphs, tables and diagrams to enable physiotherapy, occupational therapy students and readers to grasp real mechanisms that is essential for safe pediatric rehabilitation practice. Dr.Azzam sincerely hope that your reading of pediatric rehabilitation and occupational therapy books not only profitable to you but also stimulate your permenant interest in the fascinating subject of physiotherapy.

145

Printed in the United States
By Bookmasters